D0518059

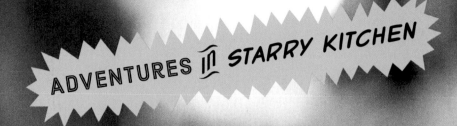

ADVENTURES IN STARRY KITCHEN

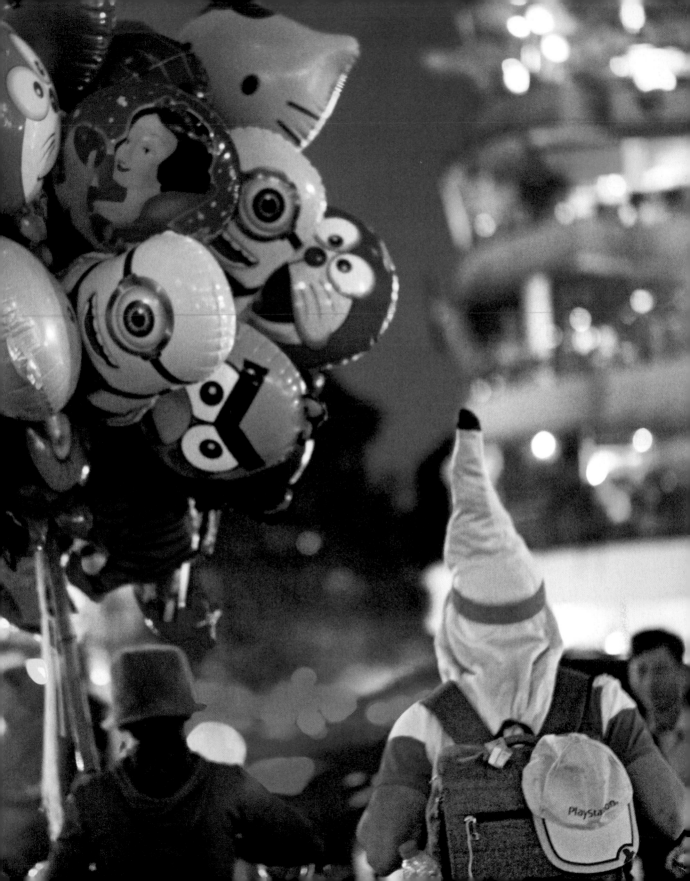

ADVENTURES IN STARRY KITCHEN

NGUYEN TRAN

88 ASIAN-INSPIRED RECIPES
FROM
AMERICA'S MOST FAMOUS UNDERGROUND RESTAURANT

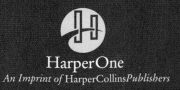

HarperOne
An Imprint of HarperCollinsPublishers

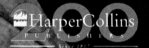

All photographs by Bao Minh Nguyen, except those on pages 2, 5, 108 (by the author); page 29 (by Peter "The Offalo" Cheng); and page 109, courtesy of the *Los Angeles Times*.

HarperCollins books may be purchased for educational, busi-ness, or sales promotional use. For information, please email the Special Markets Department at SPsales@harpercollins.com.

FIRST EDITION

Book design by Shubhani Sarkar, sarkardesignstudio.com
Illustrations by Joseph Harmon

Library of Congress Cataloging-in-Publication Data is available upon request.

ISBN 978-0-06-243854-6

17 18 19 20 21 LSC 10 9 8 7 6 5 4 3 2 1

TO EVERY SINGLE SOUL
WHO HELPED MAKE
STARRY KITCHEN A REALITY
AND TO CILLÍAN, BY FAR THE
BEST THING I EVER MADE.
WORK HARD, PLAY HARD,
AND KARAOKE.

CONTENTS

Introduction ix

FUNEMPLOYMENT

BASIC RECIPES

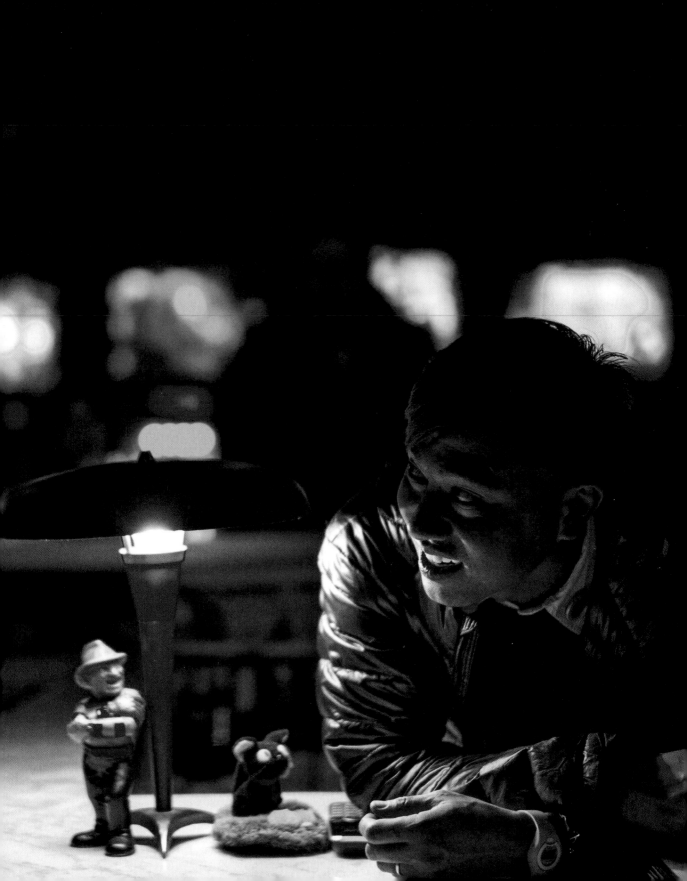

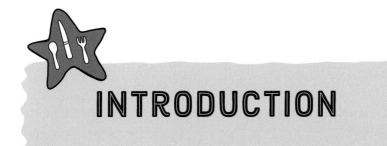

INTRODUCTION

HI, I'M NGUYEN. I'M NO ONE SPECIAL.

I MEAN, I'M JUST A VIETNAMESE-AMERICAN "KID" WITH A MOM AND DAD WHO LEFT THEIR HOMELAND AT THE END OF THE VIETNAM WAR AT THE RESPECTIVE AGES OF SIXTEEN AND SEVENTEEN, CAME TO THE STATES, GOT KNOCKED UP, HAD A KID WHO WAS A PICKY EATER (ME), MOVED TO THE GREAT STATE OF TEXAS, GAVE BIRTH TO MY MUCH MORE ARTISTICALLY TALENTED YOUNGER SISTER VIVIEN (NOT ME), AND WORKED NEARLY AROUND THE CLOCK MANAGING LOCAL 7-ELEVENS TO AFFORD US A BETTER LIFE.

I (barely) grew up on chips and queso, hamburgers and hot dogs, and other kinds of standard American fare (T.G.I. Friday's chicken fingers and their long-forgotten creole mustard are still my JAM. Ohhhhh yes!). I resisted eating Vietnamese food because I couldn't understand being "just Vietnamese" growing up (the diaspora dilemma). In a magazine interview, my mom threw me under the Vietnamese heritage bus and told them I ate only burgers and hotdogs, and I was constantly bullied for being a "Chinese kid" (those kids are more educated, know better now, and I'm even friends with some—my contribution to society). I went to college locally where I stuck to delusions of being a doctor, so much so that I even took the notorious eight-hour medical school entrance exam, the MCAT, during which I realized I didn't want to be a doctor and proceeded to take the best and most influential nap of my life.

All that time, I never thought about how food played such an integral part in my life. My first job was as a bag boy at a grocery store; my after–high school hangout was my friend's Indian restaurant (and the buffet line was subsequently my "study area of preference"); and my big dream as a kid was to host and pay for a dinner in a luxurious revolving ballroom restaurant like the one at the top of Reunion Tower in Dallas for ALL my friends. I used to eat like a football player, and my favorite personal sport was to see how many Thanksgiving dinners I could squeeze into one day (I believe five was my record—no amount of tryptophan is gonna put me DOWN!). A dot.com job gave this doe-eyed twenty-one-year-old kid a personal expense account that grew to nearly $25k per month, which became my fine dining and wine education (but not much wine because my tolerance for alcohol is laughably low), and I surf more food porn than any straight man should ever admit to (I can't help it, there's so much of it).

To put it simply: I love food.

Let's level with each other here right from the start. I am literally the biggest fuckup I KNOW! I have friends who are far more successful, make more money, have seen more of the world, and have contributed much more to society than I have. But recently I figured out that I have one God (or similar deity)–given talent: I am stupid enough not to give a flying fuck about anyone's opinion. And when I have my mind set on something, I try over and over and over again until I succeed, prove people's opinions wrong (the greatest fuel to my man-child-like drive), or—on the not-so-rare occasion when I fail and fall on my face— look like the biggest fool trying. My soul begs for completion, and begs to see if an idea really is as idiotic as people think it is. That's the best way I can describe . . . the one thing I am best at.

This realization didn't become evident until I accidentally delved into the restaurant business with my wife, Thi, my Kitchen Ninja and Starry Kitchen's not-so-secret weapon. Calling my profession an accident may sound unappreciative (and it's not meant to because I have so much respect for *all* small business owners), but owning a restaurant wasn't our original dream. But it made sense as the next step of a far-fetched idea, born out of unemployment, about running an underground and definitely illegal restaurant out of our tiny apartment in North Hollywood, California, right in the heart of Los Angeles's infamous (San Fernando) Valley.

Back in the mid-aughts, Thi started cooking all sorts of fantastical Asian dishes, taking pictures of them and posting them on Facebook. (This was pre-#foodpornrevolution, and when taking pictures of food [with film] was still wholly owned by Asians—but not anymore.)

Then in 2008 the economy went to shit. Thi lost her job in advertising the next year and vented on Facebook about finding another job in advertising, as one does. The response was unanimous: "Advertising? *Pffft!* YOU SHOULD COOK!" After about two months of cajoling and finally coercion, we hosted our first lunch service out of our tiny apartment.

We flyered three hundred apartments in our building and advertised on Facebook our "restaurant," which we called Starry Kitchen. We debated the name for no longer than . . . one minute, and named it after Thi's favorite Cantonese cooking show at the time on the TVB television network from Hong Kong (drop this on any Cantonese-speaking person in the free world, and you'll get instant street cred), which we knew we'd be stuck with if whatever this would become worked.

It wasn't fancy. We buzzed guests in, directed them to take the elevator upstairs, then set them up on our communal patio shared with other residents (and future Starry Kitchen confidants) full of random chairs in the middle of a concrete high-rise paradise. I sat at a little folding table with a printed picture of our dog and mascot, GQ (who was more recognizable and well known than we personally were in our complex), taped to the front of the table, and took orders for plates of Thi's version of Asian comfort food directly influenced by the Kogi revolution happening in LA at the time—such as Vietnamese *Thit Kho* (braised coconut pork) or Korean *kalbijim* (braised Korean short rib stew). There was a suggested $5 donation, and after guests voluntarily dropped money in the box (I never touched it) I yelled the order back into the apartment—like at your favorite greasy-spoon diner. Our friends came out to support us (we knew we could guilt them all into at least one meal). But then, surprisingly they liked it! In fact, they loved it. And those friends brought friends, and friends of their friends brought more friends.

The party grew so much that we added a Wednesday "dinner service." Yelp reviews began to pop up, which brought in even more people. Our patrons were pretty random, but my favorite group was the game developers, dominated by my small cadre of friends who had graduated from Carnegie Mellon. If anyone was the catalyst for our explosion, it was them. Suddenly, our apartment became the No. 1 Asian fusion "restaurant" listing in all of LA on Yelp.

Then, *LA Weekly* found us, which brought us patrons from San Francisco and New York City. As we began to receive more press, we got even bigger—big enough that the health department found us.

But even when the health department thought they had us, I was already in negotiations to take Starry Kitchen into a real establishment with proper permits. I offered myself to become their poster child—*Illegal Restaurant Goes Legit*—but they didn't care and gave us a verbal slap-on-the-wrist warning to shut down instead. (We didn't.)

For the next three months, we operated Starry Kitchen in "black-ops mode" behind closed doors until we finally locked down a former sushi joint in downtown LA where we could finally serve lunch to hungry workers out in the open as a regular . . . restaurant! On our last night in our apartment, we invited everyone, and 130+ people came into our home for our most popular dish, our infamous Crispy Tofu Balls. Everyone wished us farewell from the underground into the world of legitimacy.

It's been over seven years since we began Starry Kitchen in our apartment. But it feels like we've been in this business our entire lives. It's amazing to think how far we've come from turning an illegal dinner party into a full-blown lunch restaurant, closing that restaurant down, then reinventing ourselves three times, not including the numerous side "quest" projects we blindly try because I guess I get bored. Rather than looking for new jobs or staying put in the ones that didn't satisfy us, which we probably should have done, we walked down the road less traveled—a torturously unbeaten path paved with metal-screw-made salads, working in two inches of sludgy water, crab-claw-cut cuticles, and, most consistently, being broke through the process. Not just the path of owning a restaurant, but the pursuit of a concept and idea so deceptively simple I now understand why most people are reticent to admit it's even possible—to do what you love and to make a living doing what you love.

It still surprises me when people tell me how much the Starry Kitchen story resonates

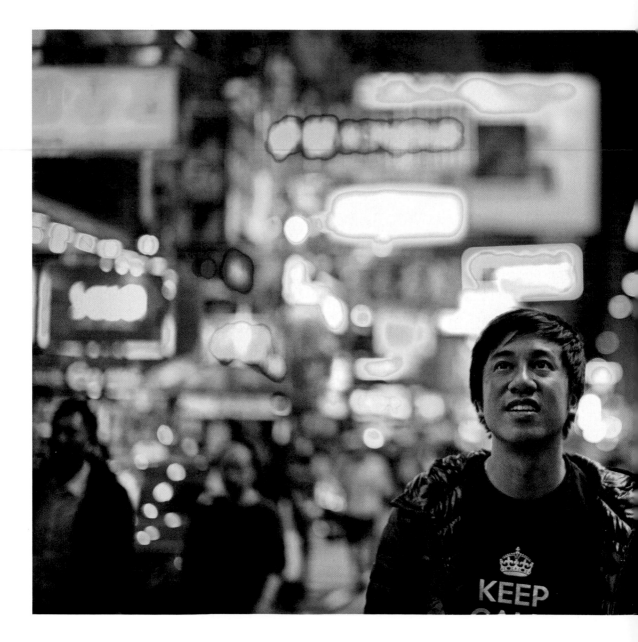

with them—kind of like how the original popularity of our underground restaurant initially surprised me. I understood that our friends and neighbors would love the idea and the food, but the fact that it attracted strangers from all over the country amazes me to this day. But the older and wiser I get, the more I understand why our story speaks to so many people. It speaks to people because it's a great representation of the proud American tradition of not giving a fuck and going balls-out.

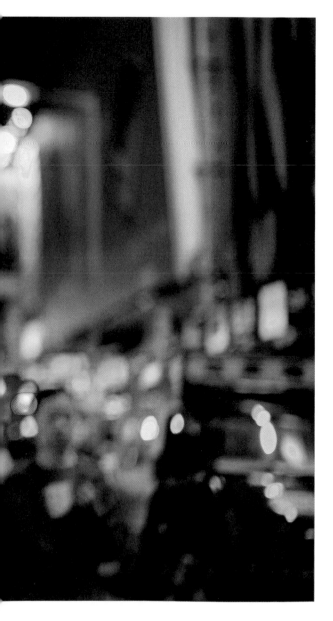

What follows is the true story of Starry Kitchen, all of our illegal and extracurricular culinary adventures that inspire the food we make—told through anecdotes and tall tales—and chock-full of drool-inducing recipes with as much food porn as these pages can hold, spanning the Asian food spectrum (and some not-so-Asian dishes because we're American, too, dammit!). Every recipe has a story, particularly for us. Stories about how we spawned a restaurant, a brand, and a stream of pop-ups and brick-and-mortar successes and (many) failures that wouldn't exist without the recipes that earned us coverage in the *New York Times*, the *New Yorker*, *Food & Wine*, NPR, Vice's *Munchies*, the Cooking Channel, and more.

They are a celebration of our food, our culture, and our personality, and a reflection of how mind-blowingly more delicious food simply is once you learn the context and soul behind it. When we ran Starry Kitchen out of our apartment, my job was the front of house, host, storyteller. While Thi cooked, I entertained guests with the story of all the events of Starry Kitchen's evolution and all of the events that transpired as we were living it, and as we (scarily) continue to live it now, through the inspiration, harrowing conflicts, tremendous triumphs, and all the miraculous support we don't deserve and have had. We're living the next unknown chapter of our lives.

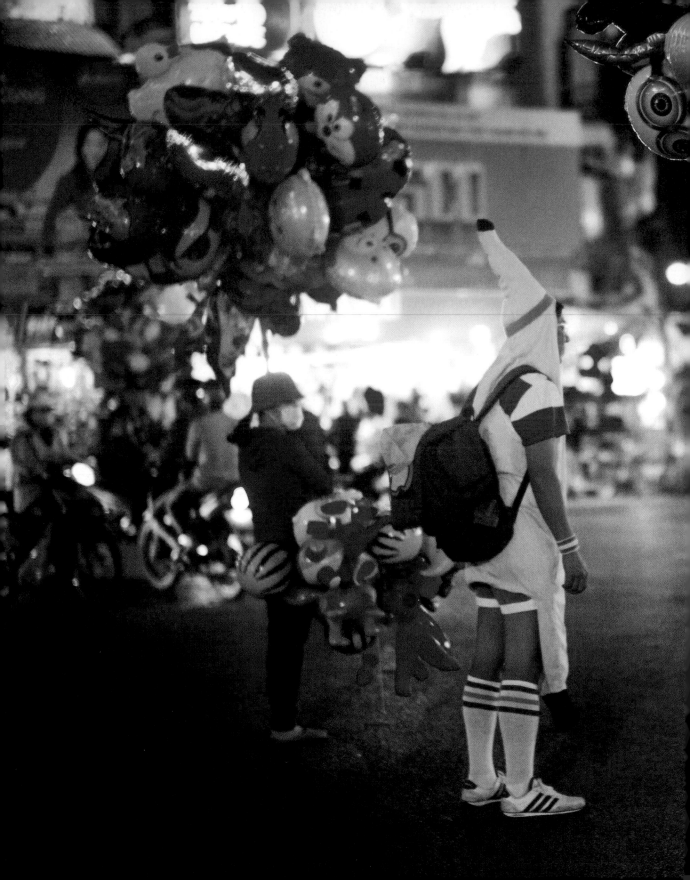

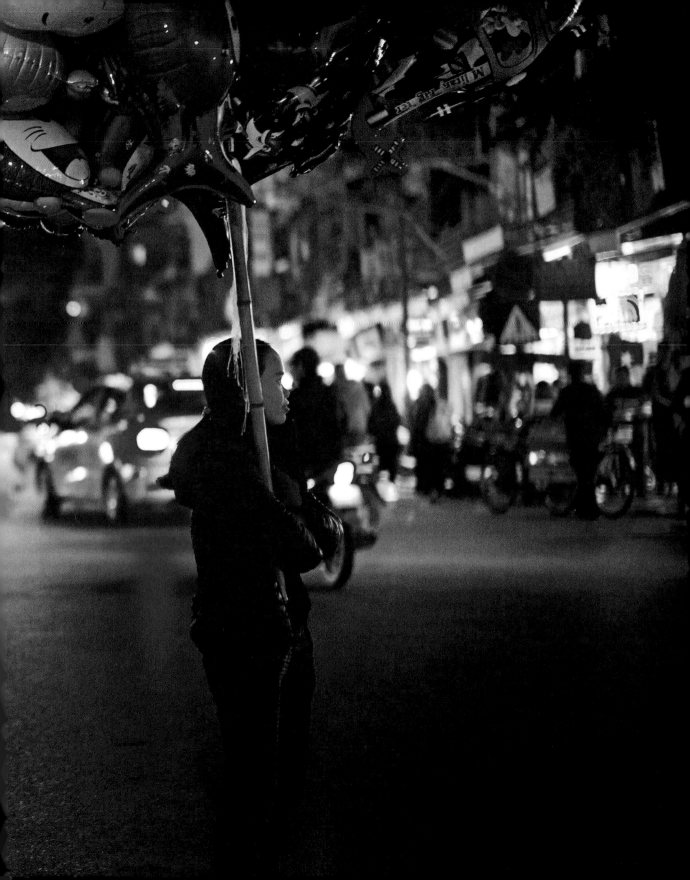

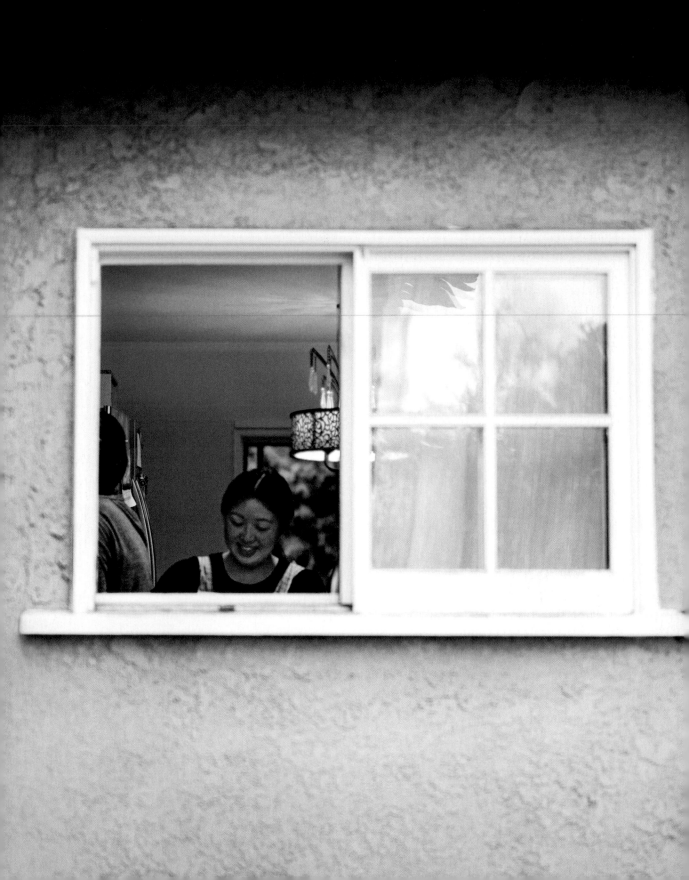

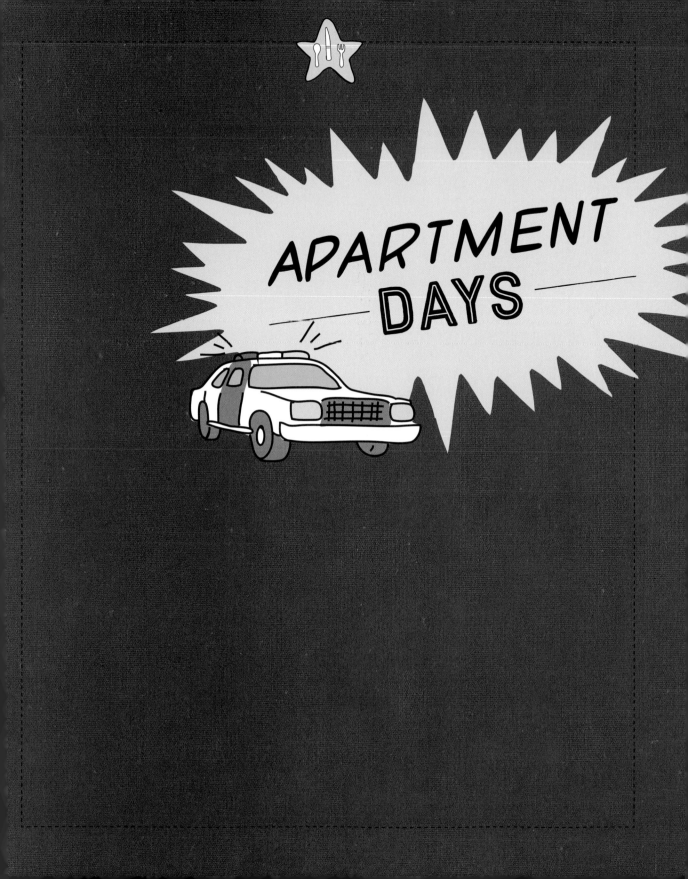

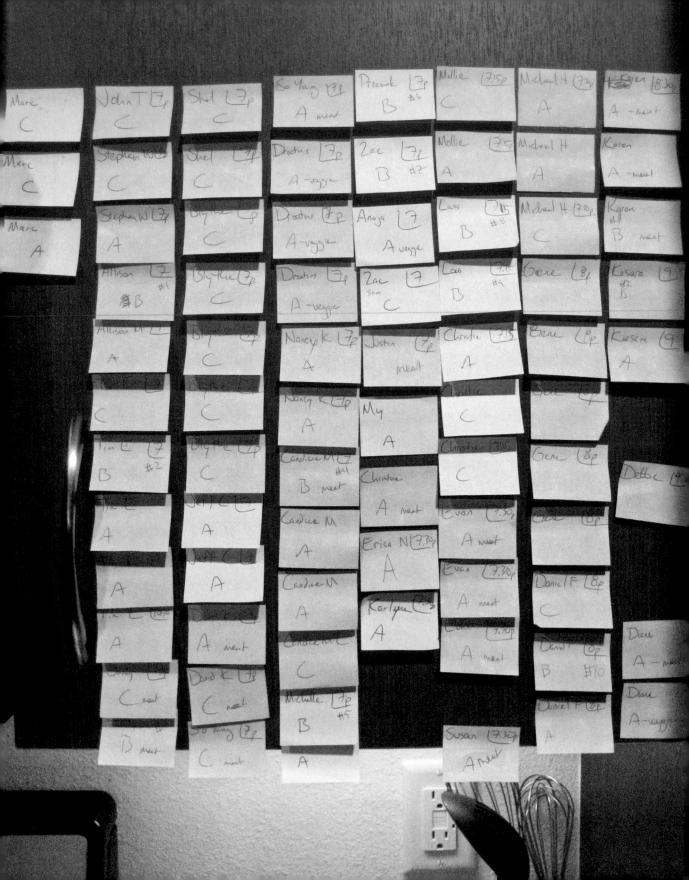

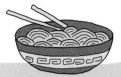

THE RESTAURANT IN APARTMENT NO. 205

ONE MONTH INTO OUR UNDERGROUND LUNCH OPERATION OUT OF OUR APARTMENT, THI AND I WERE GETTING SO BUSY WE EXPANDED OUR "SERVICE" FROM SUNDAY LUNCH TO INCLUDE WEDNESDAY DINNERS. OUR FRIEND ALEX OW, FORMER EXECUTIVE CHEF OF THE BEVERLY HILLS HOTEL, GAVE US THE MOST OBSERVANT PIECE OF ADVICE THAT REALLY RANG TRUE FOR ALL THE ILLEGAL+UNDERGROUND DAYS: "YOU'RE GOING TO RUN OUT OF ROOM FAST." AND WE DID; WE COULD HANDLE ONLY TWO MEALS A WEEK. BUT IT WAS ALSO THE VOLUME. SOMETIMES IT WAS MANIC—FOR A LITTLE APARTMENT RESTAURANT OR A NORMAL SMALL RESTAURANT. WE WERE FLOODED WITH PEOPLE WHO WANTED TO BE PART OF OUR LITTLE STORY.

We built up our "regulars." Which was great, but the newcomers, who always arrived after the regulars, sometimes got screwed because we'd run out of food. People would tell us, "That's a good problem to have," but by then people's enthusiastic expectations were starting to teeter into soul-crushing disappointment. It's horrible to be on the "piss-ee" side when people are . . . pissed.

So we started instituting a reservation system of sorts. We would stage people out in increments of fifteen minutes over the course of three hours, taking their orders and quantities beforehand, which allowed us to keep up a consistent output. At times, we would have between fifty and seventy preorders before we even "opened" our doors. None of this was expected.

As we continued to receive more and more press, more and more people showed up, turning into enough press and people to attract the attention of the health department. One afternoon, I came home to find an inspector's business card waiting for me on our welcome mat. This was the moment I had been waiting for. This is how I knew we had made it. And even if money wasn't exploding from our couches and mattresses yet, it was the moment that we were going to exploit to the motherfucking fullest.

When I called the health department, the first thing the woman on the phone asked me was whether we had a kitchen at our "establishment," and I was like, "Yeah, it's an apartment." And then she got to the real point (of attack) and accused me of running an illegal operation out of our apartment. That's when I got philosophical on her ass and asked her what the difference was between having a dinner party and running a restaurant. My contention was that this happened to be a dinner party of friends who also brought more friends, and we asked people to make donations to cover our costs.

Knowing that the health department wouldn't take this conversation lightly, I blasted out to our mailing list of about six hundred that we were finally on the department's radar. My message also included strict instructions on what to do if health department officials showed up during one of our services. The basic plan involved me swinging the front door wide open and everyone yelling out in unison, "Hello FRIENDS!" because that's what you do when you're hosting a "dinner party."

On the first night right after I called and spoke to the health department, while Thi and I were waiting for the guests to arrive, two health department agents showed up, flashing their badges. "I don't think you want us to come in," one said when I invited them into our empty apartment. I graciously began whittling them away with my obnoxious brand of kindness: "No problem, we're hosting a dinner party and would love for you guys to join us." And then, our game of Keyser Söze–like cat and mouse began.

The two agents started interrogating me, and I asked whether they wanted anything to eat. They declined, but I could see the younger of the two crack a slight smile—he was more interested and hungry than he knew. I can't blame the guy, especially with the scent of *kalbi-chim* (Korean braised beef short ribs) filling the air with all its savory sweetness, its unadulterated Korean amazingness. Like Lynda Carter / Wonder Woman deflecting bullets with her wristbands, however, these guys ignored my invitation to dine and continued their interrogation.

"You're running an illegal operation," one of them said.

"What?" I replied. "I never thought about it like that. Interesting!"

"You're taking money for your food."

"We're taking *donations,*" I corrected them. This was 100 percent true. I always put out a donation box on the opposite end of the apartment, far away from me and Thi. We never touched it. People put in however much they wanted or didn't want to put in. Money never exchanged hands.

> Two health department agents showed up, flashing their badges. "I don't think you want us to come in . . ."

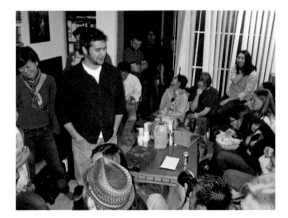

"Sir, you're operating a business."

"No, sir, I'm not. I'm running a dinner party that everyone's invited to. If I were running a business, I would have the right to refuse anyone's business. If it's a donation-based effort, it's the exact opposite. Anyone, and I mean ANYONE, is allowed to take our offerings with or without offering anything in return."

The older agent, who was clearly wiser than his younger partner, asked, "So ANYONE can come in?"

"Yes?" I answered, shrugging my shoulders in what I hoped he took as a sign of youthful ignorance rather than a tacit admission of guilt, which I'm pretty sure it was.

"You have signage on the street."

"No, we don't. You're making that up."

Why on earth would I want to advertise our illegal operation with signage? The entire appeal of Starry Kitchen, other than the food, of course, was the fact that it was hard to find, that it was underground.

The conversation went back and forth like this for a while. In the meantime, Thi was moving in and out of the kitchen, steaming.

She was LIVID. I mean, the air in the room changed. It was like one of those Dragon Ball Z moments where her anger ignited the air around us, and you could feel the hatred from across continents, it was so strong. I think I was more scared of her than of the health department guys. Yeah, she was *scary*!

The agents would present a new argument, and I'd give them my weasel way out of that angle until . . . whoa ho HO, UNTIL they dropped a pretty clever bomb on me that completely caught me by surprise.

When the older agent asked how I invited people over, I told them it was just word of mouth . . . and then . . . and THEN they presented me with a printout of my ENTIRE TWITTER FEED, which advertised the time and place of ALL of our "services!" (High-five and well-played, health department!) I did NOT expect that one, ESPECIALLY because I knew everything I was tweeting. These tweets were public calls to anyone listening, retweeting, and the like to come on over . . . and partake in the illegalness that was our humble little . . . illegal+underground restaurant.

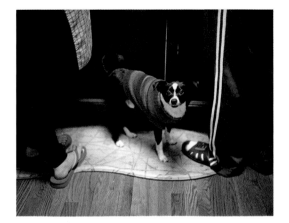

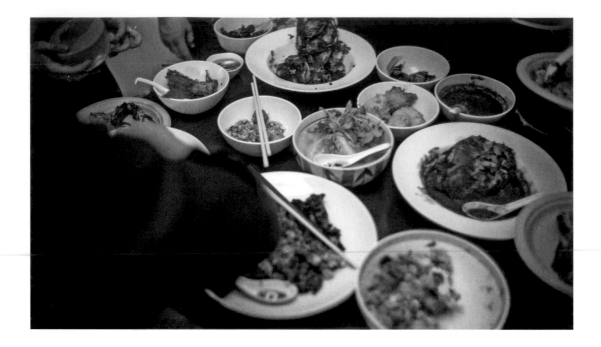

Thi put up her apron, assumed a mean resting bitch face, walked THROUGH us, and sat on the couch in the living room, arms crossed, staring straight ahead at nothingness and just looking PISSED! I carried along as if we were just having another lovers' quarrel . . . oh, to be in LOVE!

When the agents continued to press me about my tweets, I did what I saw my cute female friends do when politely declining guys' advances but getting out of them as many drinks as they could. I smugly chuckled and gave an "Oh YOU!" sigh and dismissed this printout and claim that Twitter was how I communicated with my "friends."

Amazingly, during this thirty- to forty-five-minute "conversation," not one "dinner party guest" showed up. Normally, we'd be packed to the gills at that point, full of orders, full of life,

full of youthful zest for illegal and tasty Asian street food tacos out of our home. Instead, we were (luckily) swallowed in uninterrupted silence.

After all this, and while trying to keep a big smile on my face, quietly hoping the agents would cuff me and carry me away like some kind of culinary Che Guevara, "¡*Viva Starry Kitchen*!" (for the sheer drama and hilarity of it all!), they merely told me not to do it anymore, and if they got any more calls, they'd take me to court . . . HEALTH DEPARTMENT COURT! (I didn't know that was a thing, either, if you're thinking that same thing.)

They gave me their cards, walked out, and . . . that was it! We were done in the principal's office of food service life, and we got away with it! And not ten minutes later a wave of illegal+underground regulars came in, and of

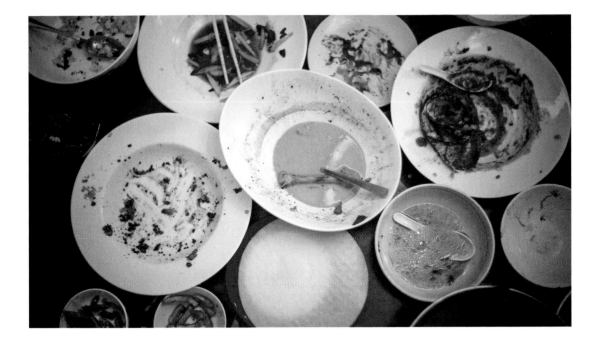

course I had to share with them the adrenaline rush of a story of what had just happened. People were amazed and in disbelief we just got away with it. It was like the moment in *Star Wars: A New Hope* at the end where they celebrate together, with awards, knowing that they MIGHT have a chance against the Evil Empire. "We did it!" All of us, celebrating together, over kalbi-*chim,* us and our unsuspecting partners, happily together in our ruse, too.

You see, I had agreed with the health department to not do it again. And knowing that the health department was smart enough to scour my social media, I had to sell the drama that we were shutting Starry Kitchen down . . . forever. We posted a goodbye blog thanking everyone, very convincingly ending Starry Kitchen. But after that, I sent a letter to everyone on the private email list telling them

that we weren't closing after all. We were just going completely black ops from here on out. Everyone was game, and I think this even more clandestine arrangement made it all even more fun and surprisingly . . . word still spread and we got bigger.

The best were emails from people who had just discovered us, saw all our postings that we were closed, and wished us well. I would reply, "What if I told you we weren't actually gone at all," which got us the best responses, and our fandom grew through this, the first Starry Kitchen historic example of how, when we gave up, we never truly gave up. But even with the 2009 Battle of the Health Department settled in Starry Kitchen's favor, we were not prepared for the ultimate war of survival as we continued to relive this crazy variably vicious cycle over and over again.

X CHICKEN STOCK ✓
X CHILI CRAB
    - BEIGNETS ☺ | MENU
☐ BLACK PEPPER CRAB | MASTER
X CHILI CRAB GUMBO ☺
- SALTED DUCK EGG CEREAL PRAWNS ✓
X CRISPY TOFU BALLS ✓
- DBL-FRIED CHIX WINGS
X ROAST PORK BELLY XO FRIED RICE
X SWEET + SOUR RIB-EYE BEEF
X VIET MINCED BEEF ✓
X MALAY CHIX ✓
- CLAYPOT STRIPED BASS ☺
X GREEN CURRY TOFU
- FISH HEADS + TAILS ☺
X SALTED PLUM LYCHEE
    PANNA COTTA ☺
(- GRILLED EGGPLANT)
- CHAYOTE, ENOKI, GUI
X PINEAPPLE BEER ✓
CHIX WING SOUP
- WATER MYLON AGUA
    FRESCA
X PICKLES!!! ✓

X BRAISED CHIX ✓
    FEET ☺
- BO LA LOT ☺
X BUN CHA HANOI
X TRES COOKED RIBS ✓
- PANDAN CHURROS
    + KAYA
- CHA CA
(X MACAU PORK)
- CHICKEN FRIED
    STEAK
- SODA CHANH
- POPIAH
- DAN DAN
X PANDAN CHICKEN ✓
X CURRY ROUX
- COOK RICE

RECIPE NOTES

IN ADDITION TO REGULAR PORTIONS, WE DECIDED TO GIVE YOU OUR ILLEGAL+ UNDERGROUND MEASUREMENTS TOO. IF YOU WANT TO HOST A BIG PARTY, START YOUR OWN UNDERGROUND CLUB, SEE WHAT ALL THE FUSS IS ABOUT, HAVE AT IT! HERE'S A QUICK NOTE ABOUT THOSE MEASUREMENTS:

"FUN SIZE" (AKA "NORMAL" PORTIONS): these singular dishes will feed about 2 to 4 people. But, because most of the dishes should be served family style, even these Fun Size portions will most likely satisfy more people. To keep it simple, make 1 dish less than the total number of guests. If you're cooking for 4 people, for instance, make at least 3 dishes and you should be good to go!

"BALLS OUT" (AKA ILLEGAL+UNDERGROUND PORTIONS): if you want to start your own illegal+underground restaurant, why guess how much to make when we've already done it. Most recipes have been multiplied to make 15x to 20x more dishes, which can accommodate about 40 to 80 guests, depending on the dishes.

Happy serving illegally+underground (and please invite us!).

BASIC INGREDIENTS AND STARRY KITCHEN RECOMMENDATIONS

ASIAN LIGHT BEER: Sapporo Light Beer, Kirin Ichiban, or Koshihikari Echigo, an awesome Japanese craft beer. Play around, get drunk, have fun!

CHICKEN BOUILLON: Lee Kum Kee brand, my wife swears by them.

CHINESE COOKING WINE: *shao shing* aka *xiao xing* aka *hua dao*.

COCO RICO BRAND SODA: a Puerto Rican brand coconut-flavored soda commonly carried in Asian grocery stores. It is kind of our secret ingredient to flavor things with just a hint of coconut but not that full coconut taste. I didn't even know it wasn't Asian until I wrote this book!

COCONUT CREAM: The Indonesian Kara brand is amazing; it will make any dish better.

COOKING OIL: Cottonseed oil, most commonly used to fry beignets, is pretty flavorless and not too oily. Because it isn't always readily available for purchase, use whatever brand you can find.

DISTILLED WHITE VINEGAR: All white vinegar from here on out is referring to 5 percent aka 50 grain. Be careful of this one characteristic. 10 percent aka 100 grain is very common, and has exactly twice the acidity and does change the flavor and outcome of what you're making . . . I mean, if you care ☺

FISH SAUCE: Super tasty Red Boat Fish Sauce is honestly the best-tasting fish sauce on the market. For economic reasons, though, we use Three Crabs Fish Sauce for volume.

LIGHT SOY SAUCE: Kikkoman or Lee Kum Kee brand.

LIME JUICE AND LEMON JUICE: Juice from fresh limes and lemons is SOOOO much better! If you don't have them, for the best flavor profile, use juices "not from concentrate."

MUSHROOM BOUILLON: Totole is our brand of choice. The bottle has a cute harmless anime mushroom on the front.

PERSIAN CUCUMBERS: not all cucumbers are created equal. Persian cucumbers, which are smaller than their pickling, hot-house cousins, are also less watery. They have a great crunch and are not overwhelmingly cucumber-y. SO DAMN GOOD!

RICE VINEGAR: Marukan brand.

SAKE: Any cheap sake or cooking sake will do, but honestly, the more expensive it is, the better it will taste . . . and the drunker you'll probably get, too, since it's so good on its own.

SALT: Starry Kitchen don't fuck with table salt. All recipes call for kosher salt.

YOUNG CHINESE MUSTARD GREENS: aka young *gai choi*, these greens are best when they're young. Slightly more bitter than normal mustard greens.

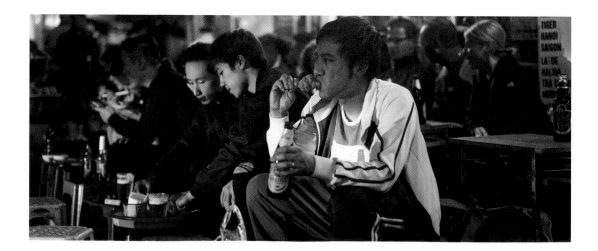

BRAISED AND CARAMELIZED VIETNAMESE COCO PORK BELLY (AKA THIT KHO)

The dish that started it all for Starry Kitchen, and THE dish every Vietnamese kid and adult in the world knows. It's incredibly savory good, and super homey.

BALLS OUT
40–80 SERVINGS

2½ cups minced shallots

60 Thai chilies, chopped

30 pounds pork belly, cut into 1-inch cubes

2½ cups fish sauce

2½ cups Caramel Sauce (page 239)

8¾ cups Coco Rico brand soda

120 soft-boiled eggs

2–4 SERVINGS

2 tablespoons minced shallots

3 whole Thai chilies, chopped

1½ pounds pork belly, cut into 1-inch cubes

2 tablespoons fish sauce

2 tablespoons Caramel Sauce (page 239)

1¾ cups Coco Rico brand soda

6 soft-boiled eggs

Scallions, chopped, for garnish

1. In a pan/wok, sauté shallots and Thai chilies with a little bit of oil over medium heat until you get some aroma in the air. When the spice in the chilies ignites, you'll know. (*cough* *cough*) Remove from heat and set aside in a small bowl.

2. In the same pan, add a little more oil, bring to high to medium-high heat. Sear and lightly brown pork belly pieces as evenly as possible. Be careful not to overcook or dry out the pork belly. This step is meant to just give the pork a little bit of color. Remove from heat and transfer to a pot.

3. Next, add previously sautéed shallots and Thai chilies to pork belly pot. Add fish sauce, Caramel Sauce, and Coco Rico soda. Mix and bring to a boil over high heat. Once the mixture boils, lower heat, cover, and let it simmer.

4. Braise for at least 1½ hours, occasionally checking pork belly for tenderness. Depending on the size of pork belly pieces, braising could take up to 3 hours (that is, the thicker you cut them, the longer it's going to take to cook them through and make them morsels juicy and "unctuous," just the way this book and we wants you to enjoy them!).

5. Remove from heat. Add soft-boiled eggs, coating each egg with the thick and savory caramel-y sauce. Let sit for 10 minutes so the eggs turn a nice dark color.

Serve over rice, garnish with scallions, and relive every Vietnamese kid's tasty youth (along with our adolescent awkwardness) with every bite.

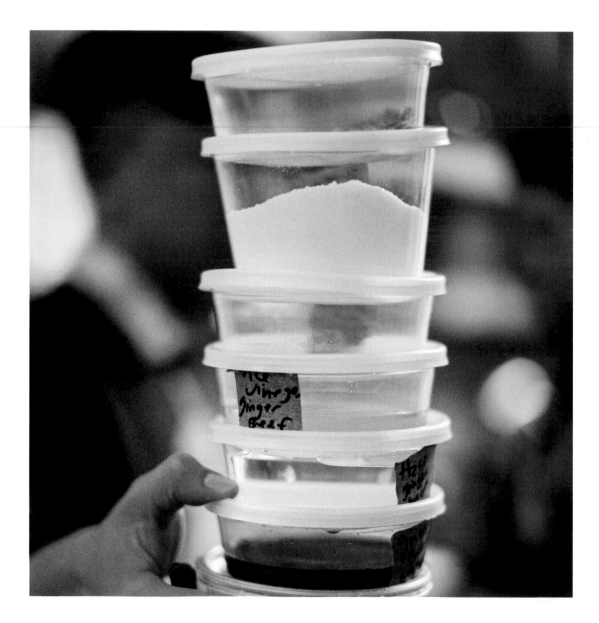

LEMONGRASS CHICKEN

There is possibly no other dish that is more palatable, more acceptable, more universally beloved, more classic . . . and more made fun of (by me) than this dish. During our rotating-menu lunch days, I would not stop making fun of people for ordering the most boring of all our dishes and the "least loved of my children." But honestly, it's fucking delicious.

BALLS OUT
40–80 SERVINGS

20 pounds dark meat chicken

1¼ cups fish sauce

5 tablespoons ground turmeric

3¾ cups minced lemongrass

40 cloves garlic, minced

60 whole Thai chilies, chopped

1¼ cups minced ginger

10 whole onions, sliced

honey, to glaze with while cooking

2–4 SERVINGS

1 pound dark meat chicken	3 tablespoons minced lemongrass	1 tablespoon minced ginger
1 tablespoon fish sauce	2 cloves garlic, minced	½ onion, sliced
¾ teaspoon ground turmeric	3 whole Thai chilies, chopped	honey, to glaze with while cooking

1. Combine chicken, fish sauce, turmeric, lemongrass, garlic, Thai chilies, and ginger in a bowl. Hand mix and massage the chicken with the marinade. Cover and refrigerate overnight to get the best flavor.

2. When ready to cook, bring a pan with a little bit of oil to medium-high heat and sauté onions for about 1 minute. Remove from heat and set aside in a bowl.

3. The chicken will taste the BEST if it can be grilled. The grill really brings out the flavor the most in the lemongrass. If grilling, bring flame to medium-high heat. Place chicken on the grill, and brush honey on the top side of the chicken. Grill for about 3–4 minutes before flipping over. Brush more honey on the chicken after flipping over.

4. If you're not grilling, just bring a pan with some cooking oil to medium-high heat, and sauté chicken for about 7–8 minutes. Brush honey on, and brush more on after flipping chicken.

   In both cases, you'll want to get a nice golden color on the chicken and cook until it's fully cooked through. Remove from heat, serve with a bed of rice and top with the onions from before. And find out why people would just ignore me even if there were more exciting options on our menu. It's pretty damn tasty.

LEMONGRASS TOFU

We have a lot of tofu tricks up our sleeves to make it taste real good, and here's a pretty damn good one, which has stuck around for more than seven years!

BALLS OUT
40–80 SERVINGS

24 blocks firm tofu, pressed and diced into ¾-inch cubes*

1½ cups sugar

3¾ cups light soy sauce

6 cups minced lemongrass†

6 tablespoons dried chili flakes

1 cup finely chopped Thai chilies

⅔ cup ground turmeric

6 tablespoons kosher salt

8 yellow or white onions, sliced

8 red bell peppers, medium diced

¾ cup minced garlic

1½ teaspoons mushroom bouillon (optional)

2–4 SERVINGS

1 block firm tofu, pressed and diced into ¾-inch cubes*

1 tablespoon sugar

2½ tablespoons light soy sauce

¼ cup minced lemongrass†

¾ teaspoon dried chili flakes

2 teaspoons finely chopped Thai chilies

1⅓ teaspoons ground turmeric

¾ teaspoon kosher salt

⅓ yellow or white onion, sliced

⅓ red bell pepper, medium diced

½ tablespoon minced garlic

1 pinch mushroom bouillon (optional)

Ginger Sesame Sake Sauce (page 242)

Fried shallots, for garnish

Scallions, chopped, for garnish

Cilantro, coarsely chopped, for garnish

Julienned Persian cucumbers, for garnish

Mint chiffonade, for garnish

Pickled Red Onions (page 249)

* Get a 19-ounce block, but if you can only get those fancy 12-ounce blocks, all ya gotta do is multiply all these measurements by 0.631578947—ya know, no big whoop ☺

† Fresh lemongrass is always better than frozen, but it's a bitch to mince, and thawed-out frozen lemongrass will do the trick.

1. See the Crispy Tofu Ball recipe (page 30) for the best way to press tofu for you. Unlike that recipe, which requires you to press tofu overnight, for this recipe, you have to press it for only 3–4 hours. Oh, and it most certainly doesn't need to be pressed as firmly, either. A light press is all that's needed to purge the surface of moisture so the tofu successfully takes in the marinade and flavor.

2. In a pot over low heat, dissolve sugar in soy sauce. Once fully dissolved, remove from heat and let it cool.

3. Combine cooled soy sauce with lemongrass, chili flakes, Thai chilies, turmeric, and salt in a bowl. Mix well.
4. Next, combine marinade with tofu in bowl for 1 hour. To get the most flavor, make sure tofu is completely covered.
5. When you're ready to eat, sauté onions in a wok/pan over medium-high heat with a little bit of oil. Toss in peppers and sauté for 1 minute before adding garlic, followed by marinated tofu. Toss and sauté those delightful cubes until they're evenly browned on most sides. Add a pinch of mushroom bouillon and Ginger Sesame Sake Sauce to taste.

Plate and garnish with shallots, scallions, cilantro, cucumbers, mint, and Pickled Red Onions. Serve with your favorite starch. Stuff your face, and eat more tofu!

She gave me more perspective
on the world in a short conversation
than I ever expected and
sent me away with inspiration.

—THE THAI PROSTITUTE WHO
INTRODUCED ME TO PANDAN/KAYA

BRAISED COCA-COLA JACKFRUIT

Most common in Indian culture, jackfruit has always fascinated us. It can take on any flavor, and when braised it pulls off of the fruit with the texture of shredded pork. It's incredibly satisfying.

BALLS OUT
40–80 SERVINGS

12 cups Coca-Cola*

12 cups water

6 cups hoisin sauce

3 cups light soy sauce

3 cups rice vinegar

¾ cup sesame oil

2¼ cups peeled and minced ginger

2 cups minced garlic

30 pounds (24 20-ounce cans) young green jackfruit in brine or water, drained

2–4 SERVINGS

1½ cups Coca-Cola*

1½ cups water

¾ cup hoisin sauce

6 tablespoons light soy sauce

6 tablespoons rice vinegar

1½ tablespoons sesame oil

4½ tablespoons peeled and minced ginger

¼ cup minced garlic

60 ounces (3 20-ounce cans) young green jackfruit in brine or water, drained

Scallions, chopped (optional)

SANDWICH-STYLE (OPTIONAL):

Sweet roll or bolillo

Starry Kitchen Mayo (page 254)

Kosher salt and pepper

Mozzarella cheese

Red onions, sliced

* Just a thought, but (pure cane sugar) Mexican Coke makes everything taste better ☺

1. Combine Coca-Cola, water, hoisin sauce, soy sauce, rice vinegar, and sesame oil in a bowl. Set aside.

2. Sauté ginger, garlic, and jackfruit with some cooking oil on medium heat. Once there's a little aroma from the ginger and garlic and you have a decent sear going on the jackfruit, add in the Coca-Cola mix.

3. Bring to a boil over high heat. Once it boils, lower heat and simmer over medium to medium-low heat. Cover and braise for about 1 hour, or until a fork can gently shred all the jackfruit, even the core. Remove from heat and let cool.

4. Once it's cooled, use your hands or forks to shred the jackfruit. Cover, refrigerate, and marinate overnight.

5. When ready to eat, reheat over medium-high heat for 7–10 minutes. Plate with rice and top with scallions, or Button Mash sandwich style. Split open a sweet roll, spread mayo on one side, add braised jackfruit, sprinkle salt and pepper, and top with mozzarella and red onions. I don't know about you, but that's one sweet vegetarian ride in a sandwich!

TAIWANESE FRIED PORK CHOP

We originally made this dish in our apartment—and it is still one of my favorites. When we went legit and served lunch, this quickly became one of the top three dishes we served over the wild 2 ½ years serving lunch in downtown Los Angeles. It's amazing as a snack, over a rice, in a Banh Mi sammie . . . I never thought I could be so sentimental about pork!

BALLS OUT
40–80 SERVINGS

40 pounds pork loin or pork chops (½-inch-thick-widthwise chops)*

1½ cups minced garlic

5 cups sake

10 cups Chinese light soy sauce

14⅓ tablespoons five-spice powder

15 cups water

40 (14-ounce) packs Chinese sweet potato starch/flour

2–4 SERVINGS

1 pound pork loin or pork chops (½-inch-thick-widthwise chops)*

1¾ teaspoons minced garlic

2 tablespoons sake

¼ cup Chinese light soy sauce

1 teaspoon five-spice powder

6 tablespoons water

1 (14-ounce) pack Chinese sweet potato starch/flour

1 bunch Thai basil, cleaned and stemmed

* When you go BIG, go pork loin—it's hella easier!

1. Use a bowl or container big enough to fit the pork, but not so big that it won't fit in your refrigerator. Add pork.
2. Combine garlic, sake, soy sauce, five-spice powder, and water in a separate bowl. Mix well.
3. Pour marinade over the pork, rubbing it into the meat. Cover and refrigerate overnight.
4. When you're ready to cook and serve the pork, fill a pot with 2 inches of oil and heat to 350°F. (Two inches may seem excessive, but if there isn't enough oil, the starch will cloud up and burn up in the oil pretty quickly, way before you can fry each chop—eventually leading to a highly unpleasant burnt batter taste and irreparable flavor damage.)
5. While waiting for oil to heat up, empty sweet potato starch into a mixing bowl. Next, coat pork with sweet potato starch by firmly pressing and then pounding the meat into the starch to make the coating stick. Because this is an eggless coating, the starch won't naturally adhere to the pork. It may seem barbaric, crude, and

rudimentary, but that's the best way to do it—a method we perfected after preparing this dish tens of thousands of times, for tens of thousands of people.

6. Once the pork is fully coated, fry for 5–7 minutes, or until it cooks through and turns a nice golden brown on both sides. Remove from pot, shake off excess oil, set aside, and let it rest.

7. Next, flash-fry basil in the same oil for no more than 5–10 seconds, or until the basil lightly crisps (but doesn't become too translucent, which is a sign it's been in the oil too long).

8. Remove from pot, shake off what you can (if you have a "spider" strainer, this will be much easier).

Serve with rice or make a really tasty Banh Mi with your fried pork, topped with flash-fried basil.

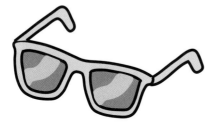

JAPANESE CURRY MEATBALLS

A friend of mine I met through Twitter—Zach Brooks aka @midtownlunchla—once told me there was no way I would ever be able to take a pretty picture of this monstrosity . . . and for the time being, he's STILL right. But it's delicious anyway.

BALLS OUT
40–80 SERVINGS

5 tablespoons ground black pepper

¾ cup plus 3 tablespoons kosher salt

3¾ tablespoons nutmeg

15 large eggs

7½ cups milk

15 cups panko

30 pounds 80–20 ground chuck

7½ yellow or white onions, minced

30 potatoes, peeled and diced into 1-inch cubes

5 pounds carrots, peeled and sliced

16¾ quarts plus ½ cup Japanese Curry Roux (page 232) or Prepackaged Curry! (page 21)

7½ onions, diced

15 ears fresh corn, off the cob

2–4 SERVINGS

1 teaspoon ground black pepper

1 tablespoon kosher salt

¼ tablespoon nutmeg

1 large egg

½ cup milk

1 cup panko

2 pounds 80–20 ground chuck

½ yellow or white onion, minced

2 potatoes, peeled and diced into 1-inch cubes

⅓ pound carrots, peeled and sliced

4½ cups Japanese Curry Roux (page 232) or Prepackaged Curry! (page 21)

½ onion, diced

1 ear fresh corn, off the cob

---

1. In a bowl, mix together black pepper, salt, and nutmeg, which helps evenly distribute dry spices later in the process—a nice trick we picked up in our not-so-illegal-anymore days of trying to be "pros" and getting better at what we do.
2. Next, beat egg in a separate bowl. Set aside.
3. Combine milk and panko in a separate bowl large enough to hold the beef. Add ground beef, minced onions, and egg and combine with dry spice mix. Mix as evenly as possible.
4. Form large meatballs about 2 to 3 inches in diameter. Set aside on a tray.
5. Set up a bowl with an ice water bath.
6. In a pot, boil 3 inches of water on high heat. Add potatoes and boil for 5–7 minutes, or until cooked through but still firm. Once cooked, remove potatoes from pot and shock in ice water bath for 2 minutes. Remove, shake off excess water, and transfer to a bowl. Set aside.
7. Next, add carrots and boil for 3–5 minutes, and repeat the same steps as for potatoes. Set aside with potatoes.
8. Heat curry in a pot over medium heat.

9. Heat a pan/wok with some oil over high heat and sauté onions until lightly browned. Transfer to curry. Next, sauté corn in the same pan for about 1–2 minutes until slightly cooked through. Transfer to curry pot. Then add potatoes for a quick sear, transfer to curry. Add carrots for a quick sear, then transfer to curry.

10. Next, sauté meatballs for 5–7 minutes, or until brown all around. Meatballs should be cooked partially through. Add to curry. Simmer over medium heat for 20–30 minutes.

Serve over a bed of rice, or as an oh-so-very-messy-but-incredibly-satisfying Banh Mi sandwich, just like we used to do back in our lunch days.

Well, FUCKING MAKE IT YOURSELF, NGUYEN TRAN!

—KITCHEN NINJA

PREPACKAGED CURRY!

If you haven't made our delicious Japanese Curry Roux, or just don't feel like it yet, you can use a prepackaged Japanese curry for the Japanese Curry Meatballs.

BALLS OUT

40–80 SERVINGS

15 (6.52-ounce) packages House brand Java Curry

10 Fuji apples, grated

7½ tablespoons honey

7½ tablespoons crushed chili flakes

15 quarts water

2–4 SERVINGS

1 (6.52-ounce) package House brand Java Curry

⅔ Fuji apple, grated

½ tablespoon honey

½ tablespoon crushed chili flakes

4 cups water

Add all ingredients to a pot/pan and heat over medium heat. Break up curry and mix until sauce is one consistency and there aren't any lumps. Add your choice of protein and vegetables and enjoy whatever makes you happy (and know that the Japanese Curry Roux is waiting for you whenever you get around to making it, ha-ha).

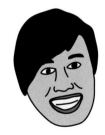

NOM NOM PORK (AKA NEM NUONG)

This dish is actually known as *nem nuong* in Vietnamese, but I renamed it Nom Nom to make it easier for (*cough* white *cough cough*) people to remember. The way we used to prepare and cut it for our lunch restaurant made it look like Spam, but it doesn't taste anything like Spam, as it's more sweetly savory. It is a traditional protein, most commonly eaten in spring rolls.

BALLS OUT
40–80 SERVINGS

10 cups sugar

3⅓ cups fish sauce

10 (2.4-ounce) packets Lobo brand nam powder*

10 pink (0.39-ounce) packets Alsa brand baking powder

10 cups whole milk

4 cups plus 3 tablespoons minced garlic

50 pounds ground pork

2–4 SERVINGS

1 cup sugar

⅓ cup fish sauce

1 (2.4-ounce) packet Lobo brand nam powder*

1 pink (0.39-ounce) packet Alsa brand baking powder

1 cup whole milk

6¾ tablespoons minced garlic

5 pounds ground pork

* The ONLY part of the Lobo brand nam package we use is the tiny packet of nam powder. We don't use the sour sausage seasoning, which is for a wholly different type of dish.

---

1. In a pan, dissolve sugar in fish sauce over low heat. Remove from heat and let cool.
2. In a bowl large enough to hold the ground pork, mix the tiny packet of nam powder, baking powder, milk, and garlic. Combine with cooled fish sauce and sugar mixture.
3. Next, mix in ground pork to marinate. This mixture will have an almost wet and loose consistency once it's fully mixed, but it should still be able to hold some form.
4. Transfer the meat to a half-size aluminum catering tray or baking pan and flatten it. Freeze for 2 hours.
5. When ready to cook, preheat oven to 350°F. Once oven is hot enough, remove pork from freezer, place tray on the middle rack of the oven, and cook for 2 hours or until fully cooked through. Pork should be pink and glistening with juices on top. To make sure the meat is done, stick it in various places with a toothpick. When pulled out, the toothpick should be clean.

6. Remove from oven and let cool for 15–20 minutes. Cut into Spam-like slices.

    When ready to eat, sear in a pan over medium-high heat until browned and lightly crispy. Because the Nom Nom *nem nuong* contains a lot of natural fat, you don't need to add oil before searing. Serve wrapped in spring rolls, over vermicelli (aka Vietnamese *bún*), in a tasty Banh Mi, or just snack on at your leisure (I do!)

Starry Kitchen speaks to people because it's a great representation of the proud American tradition of not giving a fuck and going balls out.

—INTRODUCTION

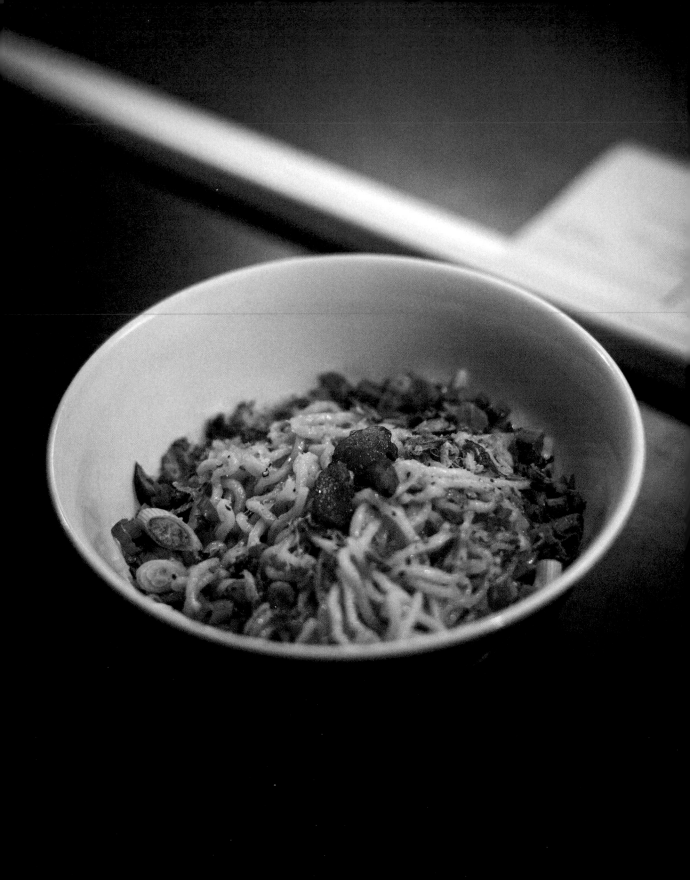

GARLIC NOODLES (AKA MAKE-OUT NOODLES!)

Since our apartment days, we've evolved this "garlicky" recipe MANY times over. Today, we marry it with schmaltz (Yiddish for chicken fat, ya didn't think I knew that, did ya?!), brown butter, and a whole lot more garlicky making-out amazingness.

2–4 SERVINGS

BALLS OUT
40–80 SERVINGS

13¾ pounds any kind of dry noodles

10 tablespoons brown butter

10 tablespoons chicken fat (schmaltz) *

1¼ cups medium-minced garlic

6⅔ tablespoons chicken bouillon

6⅔ tablespoons oyster sauce

6⅔ tablespoons fish sauce

6⅔ tablespoons sugar

2½ cups chopped scallions

2½ cups fried shallots

---

11 ounces any kind of dry noodles (spaghetti, linguini, medium-width Quon Yick brand noodles—whatever floats your boat)

½ tablespoon brown butter or clarified butter or butter

½ tablespoon chicken fat (schmaltz) *

1 tablespoon medium-minced garlic

1 teaspoon chicken bouillon

1 teaspoon oyster sauce

1 teaspoon fish sauce

1 teaspoon sugar

2 tablespoons chopped scallions

2 tablespoons fried shallots

Black pepper, coarse ground

Parmesan cheese, grated, to taste

* If you can't find and/ or are too lazy to make schmaltz, double up on the brown butter—it'll ALMOST be as good.

---

1. Since we've given a very broad choice of noodles above, let's make this clear: We prefer "al dente" noodles. I don't know what it is about people who have become so accustomed to overcooked Olive Garden–esque brainwashing about noodles and why people expect al dente at Italian places and not so much at Asian places. Tsk tsk! Get some chew. Get some bite. Chinese people invented noodles before Marco Polo brought 'em back, and it's now time to reclaim what was originally ours (or "theirs," since I'm Vietnamese) and not let Italians take all the glory for being OCD about noodles.

2. Bring a pot of water to boil over high heat. Add a pinch of salt. Once the water reaches a rolling boil, throw in noodles. Start a timer to keep track of your personal optimal noodle cooking time.

3. While the noodles cook, prepare an ice water bath in a large bowl for shocking. (If you're cooking a small batch of noodles, rinsing them in a colander with cold water is fine, too. Just make sure to run the

noodles under water until they cool completely and you can't feel any warmth in them.)

4. Stir the cooking noodles often. Get all that starch off of them. If they're thinner noodles, I would say check around the 5-minute mark and every subsequent minute after until you get a good bite on the noodles.

5. Be warned, al dente doneness with many dry noodles leaves the middle looking raw. But who cares what your eyes tell you? What do your mouth and tongue tell you? (Does it taste sexy good? Does it need to cook a little longer? Trust yourself, "use the force, Luke!")

6. Once the noodles are cooked to your liking, immediately shock them in the ice water bath for 1–2 minutes. Remove, then transfer to a colander. Quickly rinse off any remaining starch.

7. Add butter and chicken schmaltz to a pan over medium-low heat (don't burn the butter!). Brown the garlic. Then add bouillon, oyster sauce, fish sauce, and sugar. Mix until the sauce turns a uniform color.

8. Now increase to medium-high heat and add the noodles, quickly mixing, tossing, flipping your pan a bit (if you're comfortable with and good at it) to coat noodles using the heat to quickly cook that flavor in so well that the color of the sauce permeates every noodle as if the dark side of the Force has taken over and no previous rebel force colors remain (because the dark side in this case is FLAVOR!). Remove from heat and transfer to a plate.

Then do that twisty motion with your hands or tongs to make the noodles look like a chef-y pretty plate o' noodles. Garnish with chopped scallions, fried shallots, black pepper, and freshly grated parmesan cheese.

TOFU BALLS: A PRACTICE IN BEING VIETNAMESE/CANTONESE

AKA "GAME CHANGER NO. 2" AKA "THE GAME CHANGER" AKA "ONE OF THE LAST DISHES TO BE CREATED OUT OF OUR ILLEGAL+UNDERGROUND APARTMENT" THE CRISPY TOFU BALLS IS A DISH THAT DEFINES US, OUR STORY, OUR BUSINESS, AND ALMOST OUR ENTIRE HISTORY. IT'S OUR ORIGINAL SIGNATURE DISH, THE FIRST DISH PEOPLE WOULD FLOCK FAR FOR, AND THE FIRST DISH THAT MADE PEOPLE GET LIVID IF WE RAN OUT OF THEM. TO UNDERSTAND THE INCEPTION, YOU HAVE TO UNDERSTAND US . . . OKAY, MAYBE NOT US, BUT DEFINITELY MY WIFE AND GENERAL VIETNAMESE AND CANTONESE CULTURE.

Quick facts:

- The province of Canton is the closest Chinese province to Vietnam.

- More than a hundred years ago, a civil war within Canton/China drove everyone to take refuge elsewhere.

- Many of the actual "Cantonese" fled to Vietnam (and a lot of Chiu-Chow people, hence Chiu-Chow Vietnamese food, but I barely know anything about that so I'll save more for when I actually learn more); therefore, there are a LOT of Chinese-Canto-Vietnamese people in Saigon, in an area called Tra-luong.

I hate to admit it, but Vietnamese/Cantonese people always critique any food they eat, especially when they have to shell out hard-earned cash for it. The basic rule of the critique is simple: The more expensive the meal, the more passionately people critique it. The most common response at the beginning, middle, or end of a meal is, "I could make myself," which is a polite way of saying, "Why am I paying for something I could make myself?" The FACT that they could MAKE it, and make it BETTER, is all anyone at the same table needs to know.

One other rule: They'll still devour and enjoy every bite. Unless the food is actually bad. There's a very common Old World mentality of being poor, respecting food, and not wasting it, which explains why so many of my non-Asian friends are confused by Asians' voracious appetites despite their early vociferous criticism.

Okay, so now we all understand that this happens not out of disrespect but instead out of something that inherently our cultures are born with and we can't escape. So let's move on, shall we?

Simple story: Our Crispy Tofu Balls were inspired by a friend's restaurant that had tofu balls touted by a VERY well-known Food Network celebrity. After tasting them, my wife could not understand why said chef would endorse them and kept on saying to me on the way home how she could make them better and then . . . holy SHIT, she actually followed through on this motivation and DID make them better. What a lot of people don't remember is that the first version she made was with panko. Those were delicious too. But it wasn't until Thi recalled a conversation we had with my uncle Hai, who knows everything about everything—like how Tabasco sauce is best married with Vietnamese beef stew / *bo kho* (and he's TOTALLY right). He randomly suggested we try using naturally green sweet rice (*com dep xanh*) for something . . . anything. And there it was, the one element that was unique "as fuck," as the kids say. It was the "thing" that brought it all together.

The minute she introduced the sweet rice, I knew we had something very special. The response from our illegal+underground patrons was even crazier than I expected. They were floored. They couldn't believe it was tofu. It was tasty, with the texture of an egg. And it was GREEN. I mean, it took us only 50+ dishes to get there. So no big whoop. ☺

The Crispy Tofu Balls defines us, our story, our business, and almost our entire history.

〰

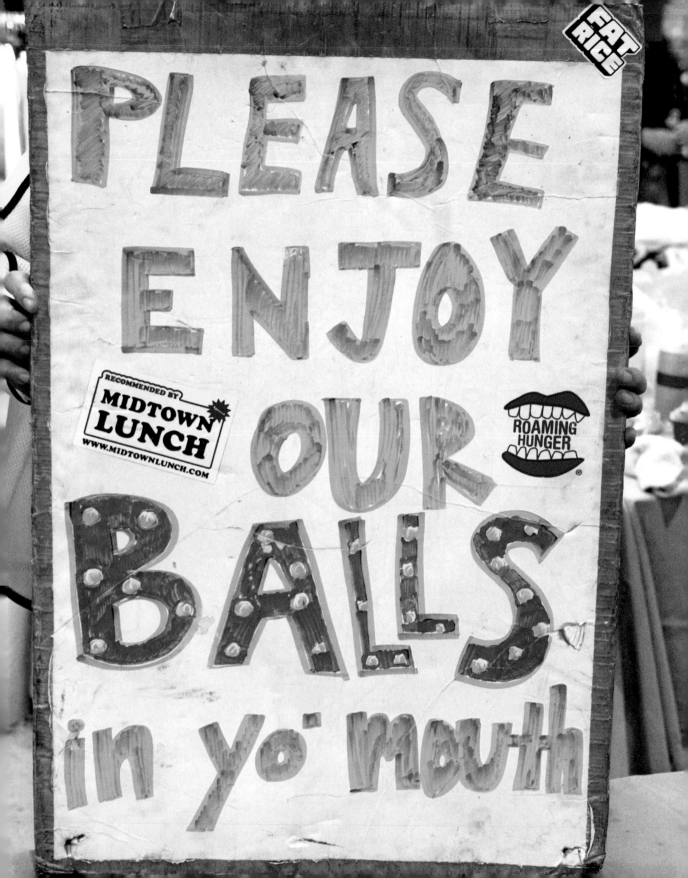

CRISPY TOFU BALLS

This dish defines Starry Kitchen and is one of the last dishes we created in our apartment. I call it the "game changer" for people who hate tofu ... deplore tofu ... cannot *stand* tofu. To get the right balance between moisture and texture, we go through a four-day process at the restaurant. For you guys, though, preparing smaller portions, you can honestly prepare the tofu day-of.

BALLS OUT

40–80 SERVINGS

24 (19-ounce) packages (two cases) firm tofu

2 quarts finely chopped scallions

2⅔ cups mushroom bouillon

6 cups fresh corn, off the cob

4 teaspoons ground white pepper

FLOUR PASTE:

6 quarts all-purpose flour

7½ quarts water

1 cup mushroom bouillon

12 (12-ounce) packages green glutinous rice flakes (aka *com dep xanh*)

6 cups cornstarch

2–4 SERVINGS

1 (19-ounce) package firm tofu

⅓ cup finely chopped scallions

5⅓ teaspoons mushroom bouillon

4 tablespoons fresh corn, off the cob

2 pinches ground white pepper

Spicy Aioli (page 253), for garnish and dip

FLOUR PASTE:

1 cup all-purpose flour

1¼ cups water

2¼ teaspoons mushroom bouillon

1 (12-ounce) package green glutinous rice flakes (aka *com dep xanh*)

½ cup cornstarch

1. **PRESS THE TOFU:** Pressing the tofu is the most important step, so I'm going to give y'all (I grew up in Texas, so I have the liberty to use "y'all" liberally) three pressing options. The first step before you press is the same: Drain the liquid from the box of tofu. *Then* press.

   (EASIEST) Use a tofu-pressing machine! I spotted one of these in Torrance, California, at a little Japanese grocery store. You place a block of tofu in between two plates and turn a small crank to compress it. Though it will press only one block at a time—the boxes of tofu we use come four to a box—you can set it and forget it (but do it three more times if you plan on using all the tofu).

   (MOST COMMON) Use two similar-size plates or relatively flat surfaces. Lay out the blocks of tofu flat in a single layer on one of the plates, and then put the second plate on top of the tofu. Press the tofu by placing at least 10 pounds of weight on top of the second plate.

   (MOST "PROFESSIONAL") We still prepare the tofu this way at our restaurant, which is, without question, the most efficient

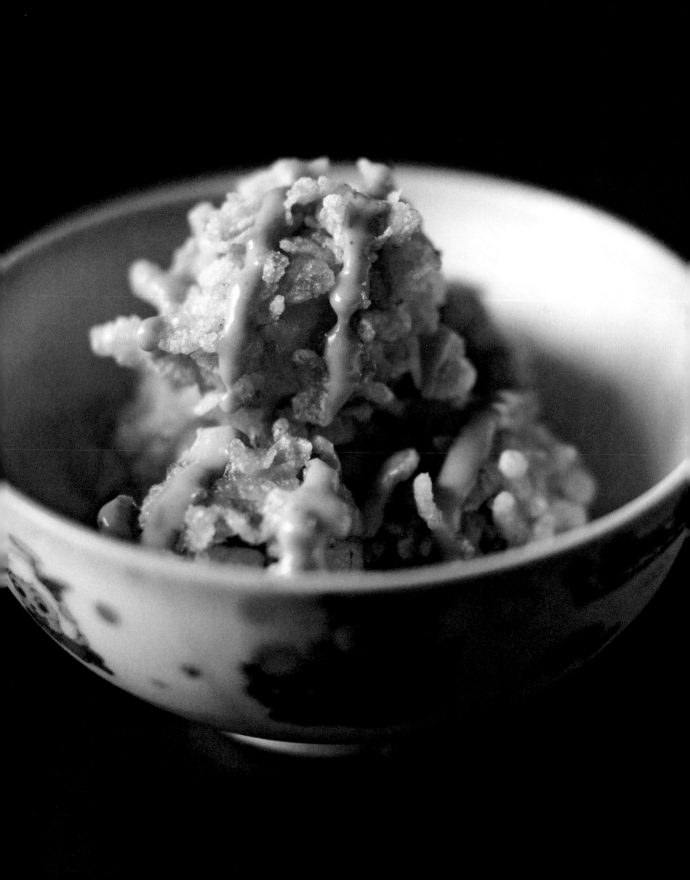

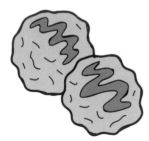

way to prepare larger servings. Lay baking racks/grates inside baking sheets, then cover racks with clean (lint-free) towels or, as we did successfully for four years, with neatly folded aprons laid in a single layer as level and as flat as possible across the racks. Yup, towels or aprons, plural. Because tofu holds so much moisture, the liquid constantly spills over, and we've found very few people who just live to clean. To absorb the moisture, and to create much less of a mess, we started using layers of cloth.

Lay out the tofu on the covered racks in a single layer, organized as tightly as possible. Make sure the tofu doesn't hang over the sides of the sheets or it won't be pressed evenly. Next, lay another towel/apron on top of the layer of tofu, again, flat and level. Then lay another equal-size baking sheet + covered rack + tofu on top of that. Repeat the same steps as needed. The top layer should be a baking sheet on which you place 30 to 40 pounds of "stuff" to press down on all the layers.

No matter how many layers you stack, the tofu should flatten out only slightly, not be completely crushed.

2. **PROCESS AND SEASON THE TOFU:** Processing the tofu is far simpler than pressing it, though like pressing, there are three different ways to do it. Start with a bowl or a large (22-quart) plastic container made by and known as a Cambro (if you have one of those lying around), and do one of the following:

USE A FOOD MILL, which is what we use. This is by far the easiest way to process tofu and get the most consistent texture (and it's a great method for mashing anything).

USE A POTATO MASHER. Just mash away, but you'll still need to use the third option to smash out any little lumps that the masher doesn't, um, well, mash.

MASH EVERYTHING WITH YOUR HANDS. (This is the most common way.)

3. Process the tofu until it is a consistent, almost pasty texture. If you go with No. 2 or No. 3, make sure to smash out all lumps from the tofu or else the seasoning won't evenly distribute throughout the mix and, later, the balls.

Add chopped scallions, mushroom bouillon, corn, and ground white pepper to the (hopefully) evenly processed tofu. Stick your hands in (maybe with gloves) and mix all the ingredients. Taste some of the mix from different areas of the bowl/container to make sure it's evenly seasoned. It should taste savory, with little bits of scallion and corn in every bite.

4. **MAKE THE TOFU BALLS:** Now it's ball-rolling time! Scoop out a tablespoon of the tofu mixture, hand-pack it tightly into the spoon, then level out the spoon with your finger. Assertively shake or scoop out the mix into your hand while mostly keeping it in one piece. Firmly clench the tofu by making a fist, packing it very tightly so it doesn't fall apart.

5. Continue by shaping into a ball, either with one hand or by lightly tossing the ball back and forth between both hands like you're playing catch with yourself. Lightly roll the tofu between your hands, moving your hands in an alternating clockwise motion, like you would forming a meatball, only more gently to smooth out any cracks. Tofu is very docile; the more you do it, the better you'll get the feel of it (like most things in life). Place tofu balls on a plate or (ideally) a baking sheet rack.

   OPTIONAL: Refrigerate the balls overnight, uncovered. This will firm them up.

6. **MAKE THE FLOUR PASTE:** Add flour, water, and mushroom bouillon to a bowl. Mix together. It should not be lumpy; the consistency should be not too thin and consistently thick enough to adhere, but not so thick it doesn't drip off your finger.

7. Empty the green rice flakes into a separate bowl or catering pan, then mix in half of the dry cornstarch with flakes. Next, drop balls into flour paste. Shake off excess paste (we highly recommend using a kitchen "spider" strainer to do this), then roll balls around in the flakes until they're fully coated. Gently clench the balls to pack one last bit of flakes onto the balls. If flakes start to drop off the balls, mix in more of the remaining cornstarch to dry flakes, then try again.

8. Set balls on a rack.

   OPTIONAL: If you plan on making more and hate waste like we do, clean and dry your hands, then sift through all the flakes. Throw out any moist clumps of flakes. Store dry flakes in a closed container, then refrigerate until your next tofu ball–rolling party!

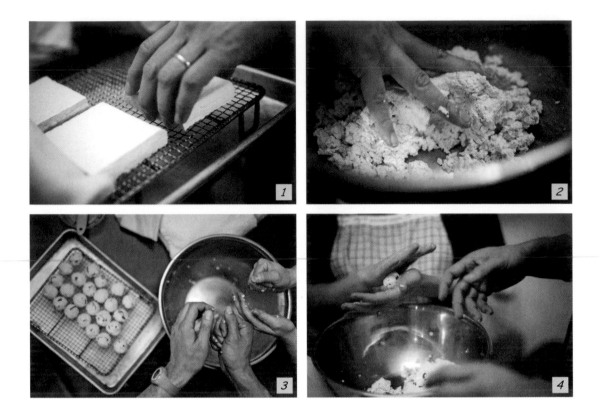

OPTIONAL: Refrigerate the fully flaked balls uncovered (and preferably elevated on a rack) overnight. This will give the flakes more time to adhere and dry out, which is important in giving the balls more puff, crunch, and an overall prettier look after frying.

9. **FRY THE TOFU BALLS:** Add at least 2 inches of oil to a pot, bring to 350°F over high heat, then fry the balls for about 3 to 4 minutes, or until the flakes puff up bright green and any exposed tofu turns a slight golden color. If the balls start turning brown, the oil's too hot or you're frying them for too long. If the balls look oily or wet after frying, either the temperature is too low or you're frying too many balls at once, which lowers the temperature of the oil too quickly.

Remove from oil, shake off excess, drip dry on a rack. Plate and top with Spicy Aioli and more aioli on the side to dip and . . . #EnjoyOurBallsinYourMouth.

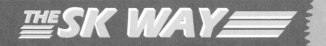

THE SK WAY

For the most consistent result when you press tofu, press overnight!

   If you're impatient or don't believe me after serving probably more than (bleep bloop bleep = my 1990s TI-85 applying complex math-e-matics) a million tofu balls by now, cool: then press for at least 3–4 hours. Excessive moisture messes with tofu's malleability factor, but we've gotten away with 3-to 4-hour presses under pressure before (for my mom in Dallas) and, "You can TOO!" (Any *Yan Can Cook* fans here? Anyone???). But 3–4 hours is the minimum.

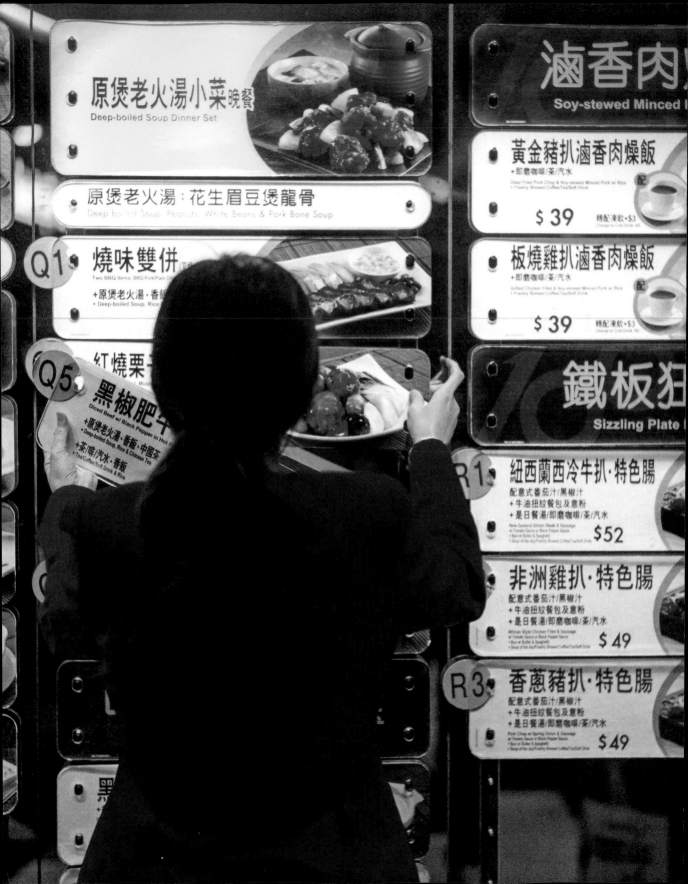

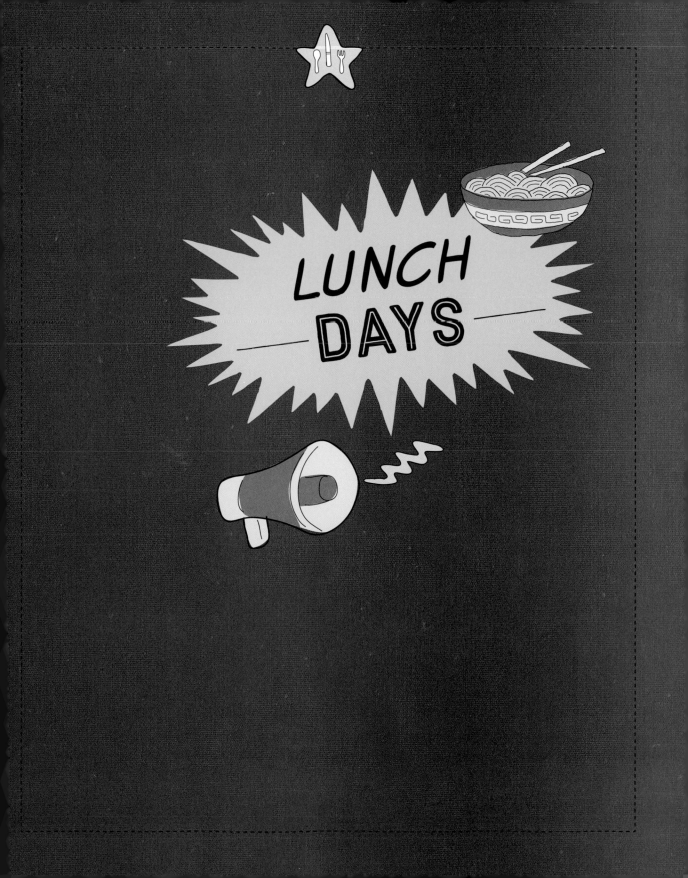

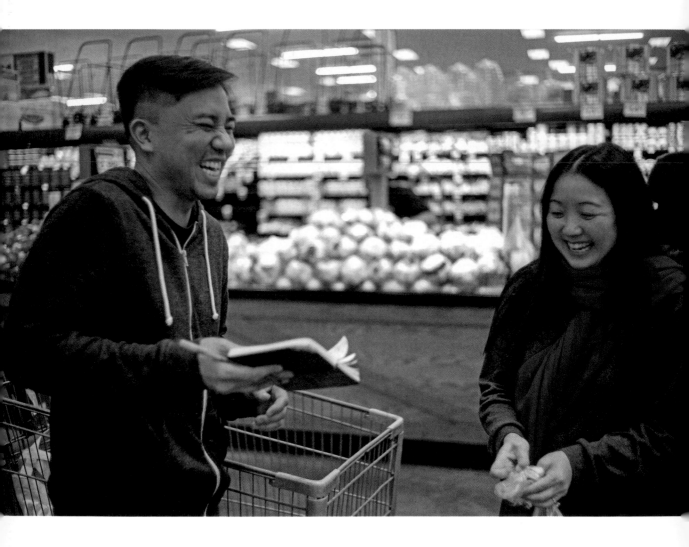

KITCHEN NINJA

MY ROLE HAS EVOLVED OVER THE HISTORY OF STARRY KITCHEN, BUT LET ME MAKE THIS ABSOLUTELY CLEAR: **MY WIFE IS THE TRUE FORCE BEHIND EVERYTHING CULINARY.** I'M HER PARTNER IN CRIME, HER RIGHT-HAND MAN. YES, I CAN AND HAVE RUN THE KITCHEN (AND STARTED RUNNING IT FULL TIME AFTER OUR 2015 RESURRECTION), BUT THE HEART, SOUL, AND TASTE OF STARRY KITCHEN—THAT'S **ALL** MY SPECIAL LADY, OUR KITCHEN NINJA, THI TRAN. I CONSULT HER ON EVERYTHING WE MAKE, EVERYTHING WE TASTE, LITERALLY ANYTHING KITCHEN-RELATED.

Thi is the first girl I ever dated who could actually cook. But fuck that misogynistic nonsense coming out of my manly mouth. Thi might be the first person I knew in my own generation who could legitimately cook well. And if I have any talent in the kitchen, it's all because of Thi, though I am definitely her worst protégé.

I figured out that Thi could cook amazing food right around the time she and I moved to California. We were living in Toluca Lake, a section of Burbank right across from the Warner Bros. movie studio. It's movie magical . . . for about the first day, and then, like everyone else, we just took the studio for granted and got used it. The first thing Thi said when we moved in was, "This kitchen is tiny." It *was* tiny, with questionably safe appliances as well. I wasn't smart enough then to understand that what Thi really meant when she said that was, "Look, I know how to fucking cook, but I'm *not* cooking in this tiny kitchen!" Which is why I cooked most of the time, usually delicious Japanese curry packets and other braises I could figure out.

We lived in that place for six years, thanks to the deal my friend Chris Smith, whom I met at a failed dot.com before, gave us. Chris owned the apartment complex, and he generously included the apartment as part of a deal for me to relocate to LA to work with him to syndicate old television shows like *Casper the Friendly Ghost* and *The Lone Ranger* to local stations. Everything was fine until the crash of 2008. Chris was forced to look at his investments, which meant he had to start charging us market value for the apartment. So we started looking for a new place to live.

Most people in Los Angeles wouldn't be caught dead in North Hollywood, but whenever Thi and I looked at places there, we kept saying the same thing: That was NIIIIIICE! Sure, there were pockets that people might call "the hood," but the places we looked at were brand spanking new. One particular space REALLY caught Thi's eye, probably because of two main features: a washer and dryer (I do NOT miss hauling my clothes to the Laundromat and back) and, the most important feature relating to our story, an open and beautifully new kitchen!

Unlike in Toluca Lake, where she hardly ever cooked, Thi couldn't *not* cook in our new place in NoHo, as the neighborhood is now called (a nickname seemingly willed into existence despite many people's objections). Before we moved, I truly thought everyone knew that Thi was a great cook. But none of our guests—including her parents and our closest friends—knew she could cook at all, let alone be close to achieving her legendary Kitchen Ninja status. I was spoiled by her meals, which meant that whenever she cooked, it was usually just for me (a nice corollary to one of my favorite rules about serving food: If you don't like it, there's more for ME!).

Once we moved to NoHo, however, the secret was out. Everyone saw another side of Thi. She suddenly started cooking all the time, and we regularly started inviting people over for dinner, which we had hardly ever done before. It was like some bizarro world where I was a victim of a wife swap . . . but with the same wife, only with a *waaaaaaaaaaaaaaaaaay* different fire and passion for food.

At this time, I was deep working in the independent film scene, traveling all over the world to help sell and produce films. Sundance, Toronto, Berlin, Cannes—you name a major film festival and I most likely attended it (unless you name Telluride . . . and Fantastic Fest . . . I haven't been to those. YET!). One of the many people I met, partied with, drank with, and, most importantly, karaoked with was my good friend June Lee, who used to work with Chan-wook Park (or Park Chan-wook, depending on how you google him), a very famous South Korean director who made some of my favorite movies, including the celebrated vengeance trilogy: *Sympathy for Mr. Vengeance, Oldboy, and Sympathy for Lady Vengeance.* June and I became such good friends that when she decided to branch off on her own to produce and adapt South Korean movies (aka "the Korean wave") in the United States, she stayed with me and Thi in LA.

This was a huge turning point in the history and inception of Starry Kitchen. If June hadn't stayed with us, we NEVER would have started Starry Kitchen. I'm sure of that. Because out of gratitude for letting her crash, and also to save money instead of going out to eat all the time, June made us traditional Korean dinners. Oh man, have I also mentioned that

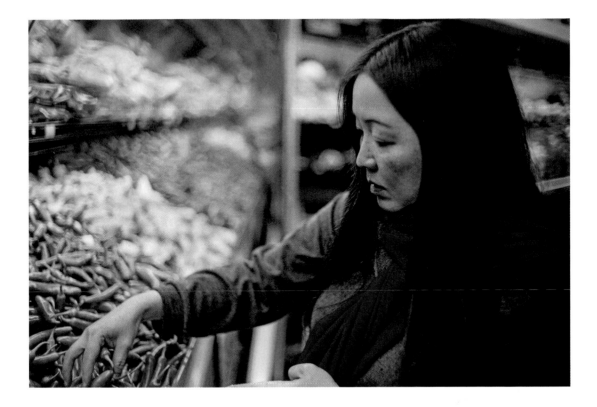

we *LUUUUUUURVE* Korean food, Koreatown . . . KOREANS?

Thi was thrilled. June introduced us to all
sorts of dishes we were familiar with but had
never seen prepared in our own home, like *kimchi chigae* (kimchi soup). We also learned about
Koreans' obsession with medium-grain rice
(which is texturally amazing. Oh man, I could
write a whole chapter about the different grains
of rice. Okay, that's not actually true, but they're
all different in your mouf—try 'em!) and . . .
I can't really remember, but there was *a lot* of
Korean cooking happening, which, of course,
led me to innocently suggest to Thi one night
that she might consider cooking more than the
go-tos of Chinese and Vietnamese food.

Thi almost flipped out on me because she
immediately assumed that I liked June's food
better than hers. But that's not what I (or most
dumb-as-me husbands) was saying at all. What
I was trying to say was that I KNEW Thi was
talented at cooking, and I thought she should
consider expanding her horizons to other
cuisines because I wanted to try *her version* of
other kinds of food.

This, as you might imagine, is a common
conversation between us. Whenever we talk
about food, Thi is always nice enough to ask
what I want her to make. And, as you've probably figured out by now, I'm not always the most
considerate man-child-like person and don't always realize (1) that I'm incredibly lucky to have

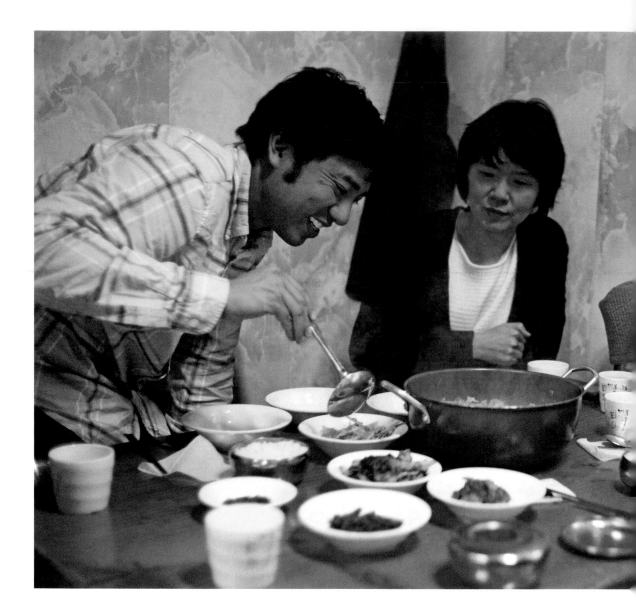

a partner in crime who can cook like a BOSS, and (2) that although she literally does ask me what I want her to make, she doesn't want to hear a laundry list of things I think she could make. Most of the time, my requests evolve from reasonable to way beyond the scope of reason.

When this happens, which is way more than I'm comfortable admitting, Thi always responds the same way: "*Well, FUCKING MAKE IT YOUR-SELF, NGUYEN TRAN!*" Which I always think is cute and a bit of a head-scratcher because, "Well, you DID ask!"

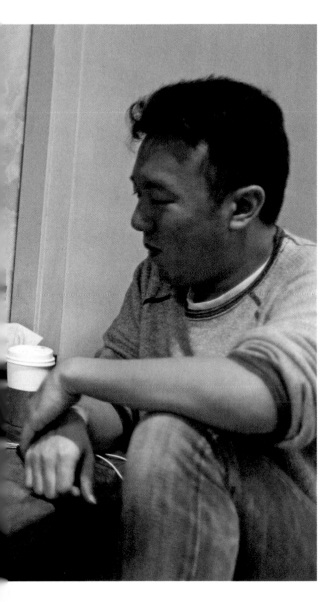

But the really funny part is knowing as much as Thi does that her reply obviously means I got under her skin—and got her thinking about how to pull off a new dish.

Anyway, when I rudely-yet-politely asked her to diversify her cooking rotation, Thi responded with the obligatory, "Why don't you fucking make it yourself, *Nguyen Tran!*" because after eight years together, this was probably the 2,555th day in a row that we had some version of this conversation. (We still have these very same conversations today.)

But, you know, I just had a strange epiphany. *Starry Kitchen Is the Ultimate Move by My Wife to Shut Me the Fuck Up!*

Holy shit. This really just came to me as I was writing about and reflecting on this. Oh man, I MUST be annoying LOL. That's really crazy to put it that way. The only problem is, I'm also like a kid when I get something I want—I want more, and I'm not afraid to ask for it, either (because who doesn't want more of a good thing?).

Within days Thi started making everything June had made for us. She started "traveling" to all sorts of countries, making dishes she had never made before and going off the deep end of food creation for nearly forty straight days—a new dish every night—and she would post pictures of ALL of these new dishes on Facebook.

She didn't post them because she aspired to be a food blogger. To understand Thi is to understand that she is mostly Asian, grew up with Chinese karaoke and Chinese films and television dramas, and is barely American. She's Asian, and Asians love taking pictures of beautiful food, and they loved it *long before* the whole wide Internet world joined the Asian food-porn order!

And before we started Starry Kitchen, that's how it all really started—so to June Lee, *We LOVE you for cooking us Korean food in our home and for making me put your food (and my foot) in my mouth one too many times!*

CUCUMBER MINT AGUA FRESCA

This recipe was born as the result of a simple comment about wasted cucumber skins, and someone suggested we make a drink out of them. Here are the refreshing results, which inspired an even more successful and smarter-than-me restaurateur to copy at his shop.

BALLS OUT
40–80 SERVINGS

20 whole (garden) cucumbers, quartered

7½ cups (13⅓ ounces) loosely packed mint leaves, cleaned

16⅔ quarts water

5 cups key lime juice

5 cups Double-concentrated simple syrup (page 138)

2–4 SERVINGS

1 whole (garden) cucumber, quartered

6 tablespoons (⅔ ounce) loosely packed mint leaves, cleaned

3¼ cups water

2 ounces key lime juice

¼ cup Double-concentrated simple syrup (refer to Watermelon Ginger Agua Fresca, page 138)

Add cucumber, mint, and however much of the water will fit in your blender (some recipes are exact; this one less so because we all have different equipment and we get it!) and then puree AWAY!

Drain into a pitcher through a chinois or fine mesh sieve. We want the essence of the cucumber, not the chunky bits. Add remaining water, lime juice, and simple syrup. Mix well. Serve immediately over ice.

HONEY SESAME DRESSING

Only after we started Starry Kitchen did I figure out that you can make your own salad dressing. Thi abhors the thought of salads, but conjured up this Honey Sesame Dressing when we realized we needed to serve salads at lunch. It's addictive like crack.

BALLS OUT

40–80 SERVINGS

5 quarts Starry Kitchen Mayo (page 254)

7½ cups rice wine vinegar

10 cups honey

5 cups sesame oil

2½ tablespoons kosher salt

Ground black pepper

2–4 SERVINGS

2 cups Starry Kitchen Mayo (page 254)

¾ cup rice wine vinegar

1 cup honey

½ cup **sesame** oil

¾ teaspoon kosher salt

Ground black pepper

Mix ingredients in a bowl, or with an immersion stick blender, if you're really fancy. Serve with slaw, salads, or as a tasty dip. We don't care. Have fun . . . and store, cover, and refrigerate when you're taking a break from having fun.

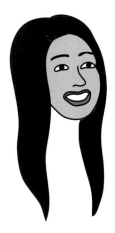

DOUBLE-FRIED CHICKEN WAAAAAAAAAAAAANGS

Try frying something right once without burning it—that's tough. Double fry it and don't fuck up—that's SCIENCE.

BALLS OUT
40–80 SERVINGS

20 pounds chicken wings*

Kosher salt and black pepper

4 quarts all-purpose flour

4 quarts cornstarch

2–4 SERVINGS

1 pound chicken wings*	1 cup all-purpose flour	* In our humble opinion, bigger wings are not always better. Less-meaty wings make the best-tasting wings.
Kosher salt and black pepper	1 cup cornstarch	

1. Season chicken wings with equal parts salt and pepper—just enough to lightly coat the wings, then rub gently into wings.

2. Mix flour and cornstarch in a mixing bowl. Dredge each wing in the mix until there's NO visible moisture on each wing. Shake off excess, then set aside on a plate or rack.

3. Pour 2 inches of oil in a pot, or enough to submerge the wings. (If you're frying up whole wings—where the drumette, the wingette, and the tip haven't been cut apart—pour in 3 inches.)

4. Over high heat, heat the oil to 350°F. Par(tially)-fry the wings for 10 minutes, then remove from pot, and shake off any excess oil. The par-fry cooks the chicken completely through, sealing in the flavor, while starting to form the outside crispy layer.

5. Set wings on a paper towel–lined plate or rack for 5 minutes, or until they cool to room temperature. This prevents the meat from over-cooking, while keeping in its moisture.

   OPTIONAL: You can store the par-fried wings in the fridge and do the second wing fry the next day. Just be sure the wings are at room temperature when you fry them.

6. Once the wings cool down, reheat the oil to 350°F and fry them a second time for 10 more minutes. The second fry crisps the wings to the point of delicious crunchiness. Remove wings, then shake off excess oil. Brush on or toss wings in a bowl with your favorite sauce

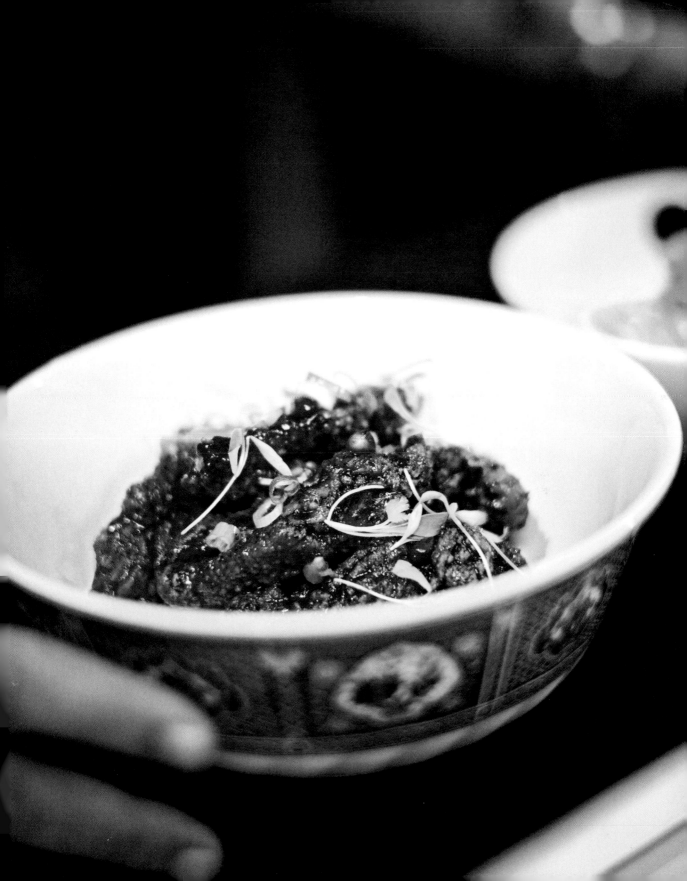

(Tamarind Wing Sauce is mine!). Or, if you just want the purest form of savory crunchy-ass wings around, eat 'em as is, which I often do as a "taste test."

7. I know I'm the stupid one out there, but when I finally realized that flavored chicken wings were just fried wings that were tossed in a sauce of your choice, I was BLOWN AWAY! I don't know how I thought wings were flavored before, but I'm also a man-child and learning about anything new blows . . . my . . . MIND! And another funny revelation: The sauces represent specific steps in Starry Kitchen's evolution:

Sweet Ginger Chicken WAAAAAAAAAAAAAAAAANG Sauce = lunch days

Tangy Korean Pepper Paste Wing Sauce = dinner pop-ups

Tamarind Wing Sauce = Button Mash

Okay, maybe no one cares that wing sauces are the purest symbolic form of our evolution (but I think it's pretty cool). So for the sheer love of all wings (and for the Internet trolls who want to take a break every now and then and just eat some Waaaaaaaaaaaaaaaaaangs), we'll include all the sauces here, together as one happy saucy family.

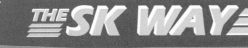

THE SK WAY

This took us about four years to figure out: If you refrigerate the wings overnight (or even two nights we just found out) after dredging them, the dredge will absorb all of the moisture, which produces the crispiest wings you can ever imagine.

If you have whole wings, cut the mid-joint so you have drumettes and wingettes + tips to serve. This will double the pieces of chicken wings you have, avoiding nuclear friend fallout when the wings run out. (That's a very scary sight, too.)

SWEET GINGER CHICKEN WAAAAAAAAAAAAAAAAANG SAUCE

Even if I have graduated on to different wing sauces, this is still my first love. I will never forget "her" (because we still serve "her" at Button Mash too) . . . oh, and this is still Thi's fave too!

BALLS OUT

40–80 SERVINGS

2½ quarts water

2½ quarts sugar

1¾ quarts rice vinegar

2½ cups light soy sauce

½ pound ginger, sliced

1 cup minced garlic

1 cup dried red chili flakes

Tapioca starch to thicken (optional)

2–4 SERVINGS

½ cup water	2½ teaspoons minced garlic	Roasted sesame seeds, for garnish
½ cup sugar	2½ teaspoons dried red chili flakes	Scallions, finely chopped, for garnish
6 tablespoons rice vinegar	Tapioca starch to thicken or cornstarch if tapioca starch isn't available (optional)	Red bell peppers, finely diced, for garnish
2 tablespoons light soy sauce		
½ ounce ginger, sliced		

1. In a pot, dissolve sugar in water over low heat. Once dissolved, mix in rice vinegar, soy sauce, ginger, garlic, and red chili flakes.

2. Simmer over low heat to reduce, or add tapioca starch to thicken the sauce more quickly to your liking. We don't like to use too much tapioca starch because it can produce an almost artificial, starchy mouth feel (which is a real term—hooray!).

Remove from heat, then sauce yo' wings up in a separate bowl tossed in sauce or brush 'em! Garnish with sesame seeds, scallions, and bell peppers.

TANGY KOREAN PEPPER PASTE WING SAUCE

This is my former favorite wing sauce and beloved pop-up wing child. It might be the prettiest of all of them too . . . but to be honest, I love wings, and I love ALL my sauces as if they were my own (which they are! ☺).

BALLS OUT
40–80 SERVINGS

4 cups finely chopped garlic

3 quarts light soy sauce

3 quarts Korean *gochujang* pepper paste

6 cups rice vinegar

4 cups sesame oil

16 lemons, squeezed for juice

8 cups honey

Tapioca starch to thicken (optional)

2–4 SERVINGS

⅓ cup finely chopped garlic

1 cup light soy sauce

1 cup Korean *gochujang* pepper paste

½ cup rice vinegar

⅓ cup sesame oil

1⅓ lemon(s), squeezed for juice

⅔ cup honey

Tapioca starch to thicken or cornstarch if tapioca starch isn't available (optional)

Scallions, chopped, for garnish

Cilantro, chopped, for garnish

Pickled Watermelon Rinds (page 251)

1. In a pot, mix together garlic, soy sauce, *gochujang*, rice vinegar, sesame oil, lemon, and honey over medium heat. Simmer to reduce just a bit, or add tapioca starch to thicken the sauce more quickly to your liking.
2. Remove from heat, and sauce yo' wings up in a separate bowl tossed in sauce or brush 'em!

    Plate and top with scallions and cilantro; serve with a tasty side o' crunchy Pickled Watermelon Rinds.

TAMARIND WING SAUCE

This is the most potent of the trinity of wing sauces—my favorite and the newest member of our wing-flavor family, bringing in the era of Button Mash.

BALLS OUT
40–80 SERVINGS

3¾ cups sugar

5 cups light soy sauce

2½ cups chili garlic sauce

5 cups tamarind paste

5 quarts rice vinegar

5 cups minced ginger

2½ cups honey

2½ cups ground black pepper

5 cups lemon juice

Tapioca starch to thicken (optional)

2–4 SERVINGS

3 tablespoons sugar

¼ cup light soy sauce

2 tablespoons chili garlic sauce

¼ cup tamarind paste

1 cup rice vinegar

¼ cup minced ginger

2 tablespoons honey

2 tablespoons ground black pepper

¼ cup lemon juice

Tapioca starch to thicken or cornstarch if tapioca starch isn't available (optional)

Scallions, chopped, for garnish

Toasted white sesame seeds, for garnish

Pomegranate seeds (optional)

Pickled Kohlrabi (page 246)

1. In a pot, completely dissolve sugar in soy sauce over low heat. Mix in chili garlic sauce, tamarind paste, rice vinegar, ginger, honey, black pepper, and lemon juice.
2. Simmer over low heat to reduce, or add tapioca starch to thicken the sauce more quickly to your liking, but don't use too much.
3. Remove from heat, and sauce dem wings up in a separate bowl with some sauce or brush 'em!

   Plate and top with scallions and sesame and pomegranate seeds; serve with a side of Pickled Kohlrabi.

PANDAN/GALANGAL CHICKEN

An original dish of Thailand that we cannot take credit for: juicy morsels of chicken deliciously wrapped in pandan leaves that beg to be unwrapped like Christmas presents (because you're not actually supposed to eat the leaf), but they're a whole lot tastier than a crappy holiday fruitcake, if anyone cares for my opinion. (Sorry Mom!)

BALLS OUT
40–80 SERVINGS

10 pounds dark meat chicken morsels

10 tablespoons minced shallots

10 tablespoons minced lemongrass

10 tablespoons grated galangal

1⅔ teaspoons white pepper

1¼ cups fish sauce

3⅓ tablespoons sugar

3⅓ tablespoons ground turmeric

1¼ cups honey

3⅓ tablespoons Chinese dark soy sauce

2½ pounds pandan leaves*

2–4 SERVINGS

1 pound dark meat, cut into 1-inch-cubed, chicken morsels

1 tablespoon minced shallots

1 tablespoon minced lemongrass

1 tablespoon grated galangal

½ teaspoon white pepper

2 tablespoons fish sauce

1 teaspoon sugar

1 teaspoon ground turmeric

2 tablespoons honey

1 teaspoon Chinese dark soy sauce

¼ pound pandan leaves*

Pickled Persian Cucumbers (page 248), on the side

Fresno chilies, sliced, on the side

* The fresher they are, the more malleable and less brittle, and they just smell NICE. This can be used in savory dishes, too (Hainan chicken, anyone?), and sweet dishes like Vietnamese *che ba mau* and Filipino *halo-halo*. If you can't find pandan leaves, we will weep for you, but without the leaves it becomes Galangal Chicken.

1. Combine ingredients, except chicken, pandan leaves, and pickles, in a bowl. Mix thoroughly, and then add chicken. Make sure every piece of chicken is covered in sauce, like "white on rice."

2. Cover the bowl, refrigerate, then marinate overnight. (If you're using the chicken for the Galangal Chicken Fried Rice, it's ready to go after it marinates overnight. You can also sauté the meat as-is and eat with rice, as a Banh Mi sammie, or even try some crazy Italian-Asian fusion, which we've done from time to time.)

3. After marinating chicken overnight, rinse pandan leaves, dry, and lay them out. Cut leaves one foot in length. If they're a little shorter or longer, that's fine.

4. Have toothpicks handy. Lay a leaf flat in front of you. Take a morsel of marinated chicken, place it on one end of the leaf, then roll it up and wrap the leaf around and all over the chicken, covering the chicken as much as possible, ideally so no chicken is visibly exposed. Stick a toothpick through the leaf wrapping and the middle of the chicken to hold the wrap. Repeat.

5. Next, heat 2 inches of oil in a pot to 350°F. Fry wrapped chicken morsels for 2½–3 minutes, or until the chicken is cooked through. Thicker pieces of chicken will require longer cooking. Remove, shake off excess oil, then plate.

Serve with nice sides of some mighty fine pickles and fresh Fresno chilies to munch on with every juicy morsel. Sit back, unwrap your tasty Southeast Asian delight, drink some beer, and have yourself a good tasty time.

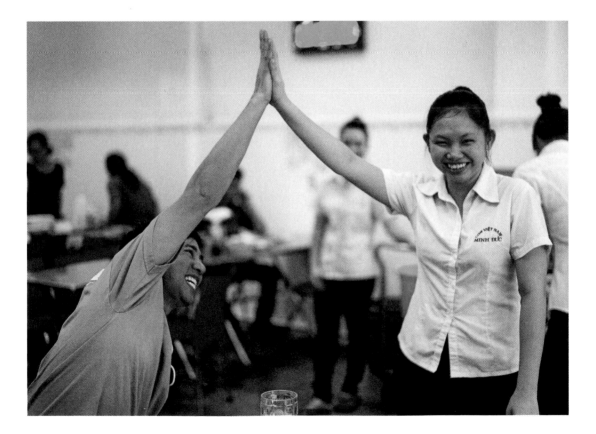

KOREAN SPICY PORK BELLY

Los Angeles has some of the BESTEST Korean food in the WORLD! And I don't mean like the world of LA; I mean in the *entire wooooorld*. The Korean-Koreans tell me this, too, but I live in LA and choose to enjoy and not debate that fact at all. We inherited this recipe from a Oaxacan worker who called himself Gordo who worked in Korean kitchens before us. We used to serve it at our lunch spot and resurrected it as a sandwich at Button Mash!

BALLS OUT

40–80 SERVINGS

20 pounds skinless pork belly, sliced*

1 cup plus 2 tablespoons light soy sauce

6⅔ tablespoons minced ginger

1¼ teaspoons ground black pepper

1½ cups plus 2⅔ tablespoons water

6½ cups Korean *gochujang* pepper paste†

3⅓ tablespoons Korean chili powder, medium coarse

1 cup plus 3 tablespoons sugar

2–4 SERVINGS

1 pound skinless pork belly; sliced Berkshire pork, aka Kurobuta pork, aka black pig, is best*

1½ tablespoons light soy sauce

1 teaspoon minced ginger

Pinch ground black pepper

1⅓ tablespoons water

5⅓ tablespoons Korean *gochujang* pepper paste†

½ tablespoon Korean chili powder, medium coarse

1 tablespoon sugar

* The easiest way to cut a slab of any meat is to partially freeze it, and then slightly thaw it out.

† Don't skimp on the *gochujang*, y'all.

1. Set aside sliced pork. Combine soy sauce, ginger, black pepper, water, *gochujang*, chili powder, and sugar in a bowl and mix. Add pork belly and massage the marinade into the meat by hand.
2. Cover and refrigerate overnight.
3. When ready to cook, grill or sauté for 3–4 minutes per side over high heat until both sides are nice and brown under all that *gochujang* red deliciousness.

   Eat it with any starch that just begs for flavor/*sabor*/SOUL . . . and share with someone you love (and feel free to be greedy and don't share with others if they aren't deserving of your love).

KARA-AGE

In short, this is Japanese popcorn chicken. Even shorter, this is better than most Super Bowl food you'll make any year.

BALLS OUT
40–80 SERVINGS

FOR PONZU DIPPING SAUCE:

8 cups light soy sauce

2⅔ cups rice vinegar

2⅔ cups mirin

½ cup bonito flakes (aka katsuobushi)

4 cups thinly julienned ginger

½ cup orange juice

KARA-AGE:

¾ cup plus 1 tablespoon minced ginger

¾ cup plus 1 tablespoon minced garlic

2½ cups sake*

1½ cups light soy sauce

5 tablespoons sugar

6⅔ tablespoons chicken bouillon

20 pounds boneless dark meat chicken, cleaned, patted dry, and cut into 1-inch morsels†

5 quarts potato starch/flour

FOR PONZU DIPPING SAUCE:

1 cup light soy sauce

⅓ cup rice vinegar

⅓ cup mirin

1 tablespoon bonito flakes (aka katsuobushi)

½ cup thinly julienned ginger

1 tablespoon orange juice

KARA-AGE:

1⅓ tablespoons minced ginger

1⅓ tablespoons minced garlic

¼ cup sake*

2½ tablespoons light soy sauce

½ tablespoon sugar

⅔ tablespoon chicken bouillon

2 pounds boneless dark meat chicken, cleaned, patted dry, and cut into 1-inch morsels†

---

2 cups potato starch/flour

Ponzu Dipping Sauce . . . for dippin'!

* Any cheap sake will do. Plus you can always play the "one for you, two for me" game while cooking with sake . . . aka just drink lots of sake while having a good time making amazing food. ☺

† Use leg or thigh meat, definitely *not* breast. Dun do it, kids!

1. Bring a pot to a simmer over medium-low heat with light soy sauce, rice vinegar, mirin, and bonito flakes. Mix well. Let it simmer for 4–5 minutes. Afterwards, remove from heat, dispose of bonito flakes, add orange juice and ginger, mix, transfer to a container, and set aside.

2. Combine ginger and garlic with sake, soy sauce, sugar, and chicken bouillon in a bowl; mix until sugar completely dissolves. If it doesn't dissolve, transfer to a pot and dissolve over low heat. Remove from heat after sugar dissolves and let cool to room temperature.

3. Next, mix chicken with marinade in a bowl. Cover and refrigerate overnight for best results, or at least 1 hour if you're just a-hankerin' for some fried chicken morseliciousness (and you're impatient and WANT IT NOW!).

4. When you're ready to cook, heat a pot with 2 inches oil to 350°F. While you're waiting for the oil to come to temperature, prepare potato starch in a separate bowl.

5. Take chicken out of marinade, shake off excess marinade, then dredge in potato starch in small enough batches to coat evenly. This is the pro move. Trust me when I say my eyes get bigger than my stomach and I just want to throw it ALL in at once. Definitely *not* a pro move. Toss in enough—not all of it. Don't be like me. Shake off excess starch. When the oil's ready, deep-fry chicken for 3–4 minutes until golden and crispy on the outside and fully cooked and still juicy on the inside.

6. Remove from oil, shake off excess oil, drip-dry on a plate with napkins, plate in a nice little bowl or on a platter, and serve with a side of ponzu dippin' sauce. SO GOOD!

Happy Super Bowl! Who cares who wins when you're snackin' on these?—because you've already won, pardner!

"CRACK" KRAB CAKES

To be honest, we didn't create this dish. Our first kitchen manager, Juve, did. It's the best example of what can happen when you give staff members a voice. Juve's dish, along with our evolution of it, became one of our All-Time Top-Three Bestsellers during our lunch days.

2–4 SERVINGS

WASABI AIOLI:

1⅓ tablespoons lemon juice

2 teaspoons sugar

⅓ teaspoon kosher salt

1⅓ tablespoons wasabi powder

1 cup Starry Kitchen Mayo (page 254)

"CRACK":

1 pound imitation crab (aka krab) meat, or real crab meat, I suppose*

⅓ teaspoon kosher salt

⅓ teaspoon ground black pepper

⅓ bunch cilantro, coarsely chopped

2 ounces jalapeños, coarsely chopped

2¼ teaspoons coarsely chopped Thai chilies

6½ tablespoon Starry Kitchen Mayo

⅔ teaspoon yuzu juice†

¹⁄₁₀ lime, zested‡

1 (2-pound) package tempura flour§

2 large eggs

1 (8-ounce) bag panko bread crumbs

* Try to find the kind of krab that actually has thin flaky strands like real crab. Try to avoid the chunky chunks, readily available everywhere.

† You can buy yuzu juice bottled. It is a little pricey, but if you have a choice of cheap versus expensive, veer toward the more expensive end. We find the cheaper ones more diluted, with less distinct flavor.

‡ Math is odd when you work backwards from a large recipe sometimes! ☺

§ Want the "good stuff"? Look for the "secret ingredient" in the tempura flour, that is, monosodium glutamate aka MSG.

BALLS OUT
40–80 SERVINGS

WASABI AIOLI:

4 cups lemon juice

2 cups sugar

6 tablespoons kosher salt

4 cups wasabi powder

12 cups Starry Kitchen Mayo (page 254)

"CRACK":

30 pounds imitation crab (aka krab) meat, or real crab meat*

3 tablespoons kosher salt

3 tablespoons ground black pepper

9 bunches cilantro, coarsely chopped

4 pounds jalapeños, coarsely chopped

1½ cups coarsely chopped Thai chilies

3 cups Starry Kitchen Mayo

6 tablespoons yuzu juice†

3 whole limes, zested‡

15 (2-pound) packages tempura flour§

30 large eggs

30 (8-ounce) bags panko bread crumbs

1. **FOR WASABI AIOLI:** Combine lemon juice, sugar, salt, and wasabi powder in a bowl. Mix until sugar dissolves. Add Starry Kitchen Mayo and fold everything together with a pleasant little spatula. Store in the fridge, and dip away!

2. **FOR THE "CRACK":** Heat 2 inches of oil in a pot to 350°F over medium-high heat.

3. Wearing gloves, combine krab, salt, black pepper, cilantro, jalapeños, Thai chilies, Starry Kitchen Mayo, yuzu juice, and lime zest in a bowl. If there was ever a time to mix like there's no tomorrow, this might be it. And while you're looking toward a tasty new tomorrow, be careful to NOT rub your eyes!

4. Next, take a small handful of your krab mix, pack it tightly together, and gently shape a Krab cake—"with a capital K," as my customers always like to remind me—about the size and shape of a hockey puck.

5. To dredge the cakes professional-like, start with three mixing bowls. In the first bowl, pour in tempura flour. In the next bowl, blend eggs. In the third bowl, pour panko bread crumbs.

6. First, lightly coat cakes all over with tempura flour. If cakes come apart, you didn't pack them well enough. Repack, recoat, and do it with more passion and fervor this time!

7. After you coat cakes with tempura flour, dredge them with eggs.

8. Finally, coat cakes with panko bread crumbs, completing the professional triple-dredge maneuver. (I'm easily amused by any cooking technique that is more than "just add water.")

9. When oil is hot, fry dem suckas, for 2 minutes per side, or until golden brown on both sides.

Remove and shake off excess oil; serve with rice or in a Banh Mi topped with Wasabi Aioli; serve with an additional side of aioli for continued wasabi delightfulness. Eat and let the crack-liciousness ensue.

MALAYSIAN CHICKEN CURRY

I love curry. ALL curries! I just do. Ours is mixed in with an Indonesian chili paste for a deep, comforting, and rich curry that will have you calling home—or maybe your Malaysian friend's home to tell her how much you miss her home. Interestingly, the best Indonesian chili paste is made in the Netherlands, where a huge Indonesian community lives. Shout out to the Indo-Dutch diaspora!

BALLS OUT
40–80 SERVINGS

3⅓ cups Yeo brand Malaysian curry powder

1 cup sugar

1 cup kosher salt

1 cup chicken bouillon

40 pounds dark meat chicken (cut, uncut, on bone, boneless—whatevs)

6 ¾ quarts coconut milk

8 cups whole milk

2 cups sambal badjak*

4 yellow or white onions, sliced

66 kaffir lime leaves, ripped in half widthwise

13⅓ pounds Okinawan sweet potatoes (aka Hawaiian purple sweet potatoes), peeled and cut into 1-inch cubes

13⅓ pounds carrots, cut into 1½-inch-long pieces

2–4 SERVINGS

1⅓ tablespoons Yeo brand Malaysian curry powder

1 teaspoon sugar

1 teaspoon kosher salt

1 teaspoon chicken bouillon

1 pound dark meat chicken (cut, uncut, bone-on, boneless—whatevs)

⅔ cup coconut milk

2⅔ tablespoons whole milk

2½ teaspoons sambal badjak*

¼ yellow or white onion, sliced

2 kaffir lime leaves, ripped in half widthwise

⅓ pound Okinawan sweet potatoes (aka Hawaiian purple sweet potatoes), peeled and cut into 1-inch cubes

⅓ pound carrots, cut into 1½-inch-long pieces

Buttermilk Beer Beignets (page 213; optional)

Scallions, coarsely chopped, for garnish

* An Indonesian chili paste with minced onions and dried shrimp.

1. Heads up, kids! The best version of this dish takes three days to make. If you have to have it now, the shortest amount of time it takes is probably 2 hours.

2. Combine curry powder, sugar, salt, and chicken bouillon in a mixing bowl and hand mix together *Sling Blade*–style ("mmmmmm hmm") until it's all one love, one mix.

3. Rinse chicken under water, pat dry with paper towels, then transfer to a mixing bowl. Next, pour the beautiful curry spice mix all over that chicken, then gently dominate that chicken. Mix and rub the spices all over the chicken until no chicken remains uncovered with spice. Cover it all up, like it's your only goal in life.

4. Marinate overnight. Alternatively, if you're in a hurry, marinate for 1 hour, though the curry mix won't fully penetrate the chicken or touch the souls of others, which is what eating is all about.

5. When ready to cook, you'll need a pan to sauté with and a pot for stewing and braising.

6. Combine coconut milk, whole milk, and sambal badjak in pot.

7. Next, heat the sauté pan to medium-high heat. Add a little bit of cooking oil, add some onions and some kaffir leaves, and sear batches of chicken until chicken turns golden brown all around, while sweating onions and leaves. Do not cook the chicken through; just brown and sear. The kaffir leaves will fill your kitchen with their incredible citrus scent—a pretty amazing smell (unless you don't like citrus, then it might be kind of annoying).

8. After each batch is evenly seared, transfer into pot. To ensure the chicken cooks evenly, do not heat up the pot until all chicken is seared. Continue searing onions, kaffir leaves, and chicken. Once all chicken is seared, sauté any remaining kaffir leaves, and onions, and transfer to the pot before cooking. If there is any excess spice mix in the chicken marinade bowl, also transfer into the pot because the spice mix is measured specifically to give the best flavor for the curry sauce itself and not just the marinade.☺

9. Bring pot to a boil over high heat, then simmer covered with a slight opening for 35–45 minutes, or until the chicken is tender but not falling apart. The curry consistency should be thin and almost milky. Once chicken is done, turn off heat.

10. While waiting for the chicken to finish cooking, prepare an ice water bath in a bowl. Bring 2 inches of water to a rolling boil in a pot over high heat. Cook the sweet potatoes in the boiling water for 6–8 minutes. Check often to see when the potatoes are cooked through; they should be crunchy, still firm and not mushy. Once they're done, remove the potatoes from pot (but do not dump the boiling water; save it for blanching the carrots) and shock them immediately in the ice water bath for 2 minutes, or until they are completely cool to the touch. Strain and set aside cooked potatoes in a fresh bowl.

11. Next, blanch the carrots by repeating the steps as for the potatoes, checking for nonmushy doneness. If you use baby carrots, they take about 4–5 minutes to blanch. Adjust time accordingly for the type of carrots you're using and how they're cut. Cook, shock, strain, then set aside with the potatoes.

12. Chicken can be served immediately, but it will be most flavorful if cooled down, stored, and covered overnight in the fridge, and then reheated and served the next day. Blanched potatoes and carrots can also be stored overnight.

13. When ready to serve (not long before—just right when you are ready to serve), add carrots and potatoes to the hot chicken curry. Garnish with scallions. Serve with steamed rice, and if you want to soak up that curry deliciousness (my favorite part), sop it up with some Buttermilk Beer Beignets.

And that's the best experience with chicken curry that you can have—reaching the epitome of chicken curry enlightenment. Enjoy, kids!

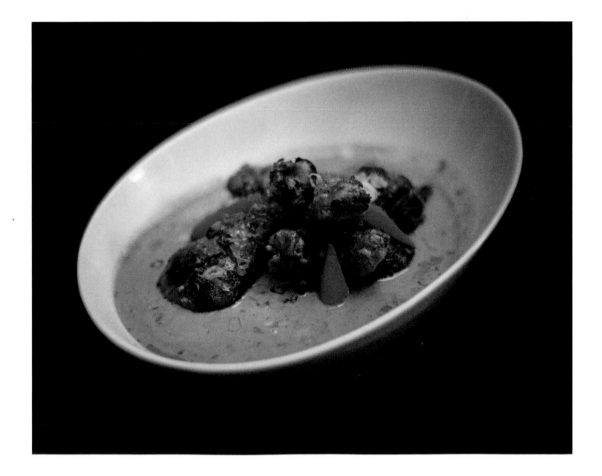

MALAYSIAN COCO CHICKEN

I'm pretty sure this dish was invented out of thin air with Malaysian flavors, random ingredients, and my "stupid" request for my wife to cook something other than Vietnamese and Chinese food. This is basically how Starry Kitchen started, too. No big deal.

BALLS OUT
40–80 SERVINGS

100 whole bay leaves

5 quarts coconut milk plus enough to cover chicken in pot

6⅔ tablespoons finely chopped Thai chilies

1¼ cups sugar

20 pounds dark meat chicken*

1¼ cups chicken bouillon

1¼ cups minced garlic

13⅓ cups sliced yellow or white onion

40 whole habañero chili peppers, sliced (optional)

4 cups pineapple tidbits, drained—as in, no liquid

2–4 SERVINGS

5 whole bay leaves

1 cup coconut milk plus enough to cover chicken in pot

⅓ tablespoon finely minced Thai chilies

1 tablespoon sugar

1 pound dark meat chicken*

1 tablespoon chicken bouillon

1 tablespoon minced garlic

⅔ cup sliced yellow or white onion

2 whole habañero chili peppers, sliced (optional)

3¼ tablespoons pineapple tidbits, drained—as in, no liquid

* Use drumsticks or boneless thigh or leg meat . . . NEVER chicken breast!

1. Combine bay leaves, coconut milk, Thai chilies, and sugar in a pot. Mix and bring to a boil over high heat. Remove from heat once sugar is completely dissolved.
2. Add a little bit of oil to a pan/wok and heat on high heat. Once it's hot, add chicken, chicken bouillon, garlic, onions, and habañero; cook until the chicken gets a nice sear and color. Be careful not to cook chicken through before braising. Also be careful if you cook with habañero, that spicy chili smell will wake you UP!
3. Now transfer chicken and sautéed vegetables to the coconut milk mix pot, and return pot to a boil. Once it boils, lower heat and simmer for 30 minutes uncovered, or until chicken is cooked through and tender. Next, mix in pineapple and immediately remove from heat and let cool. This can be eaten immediately, but we recommend you let it cool; cover and refrigerate overnight to allow the flavors to latch on to that the chicken.

    When ready to serve, reheat and serve with rice . . . or the French-Vietnamese way to eat curries and the like, with a nice fluffy loaf of French-Vietnamese bread to sop it all up with.

PINEAPPLE BEER CHICKEN WING SOUP

The trifecta of flavor: chicken wings, beer, and PINEAPPLE—kind of like the holy trinity of cooking! This was never intended to be a stand-alone dish. But Thi's mother invented it as a soup base for hotpot (*shabu-shabu*, for those more familiar with the Japanese version), basically a pot of soup that you cook in, dip, and sip at the dinner table, or eat it on its own, like me!

2–4 SERVINGS

BALLS OUT
40–80 SERVINGS

20 pounds chicken wings

20 pieces fermented bean curd (aka fermented tofu)*

6⅔ tablespoons minced garlic

6⅔ tablespoons sugar

10 tablespoons chicken bouillon

13⅓ cups fresh peeled pineapple, sliced into rings

Brown sugar, for grilling (optional)

8⅓ quarts Superconcentrated Cantonese Chicken Stock (page 256)

13⅓ tablespoons Asian light beer, plus additional for flavor

6⅔ bunches Chinese watercress

---

1 pound chicken wings

1 piece fermented bean curd (aka fermented tofu)*

⅓ tablespoon minced garlic

⅓ tablespoon sugar

½ tablespoon chicken bouillon

⅔ cup fresh peeled pineapple, sliced into rings

Brown sugar, for grilling (optional)

1⅔ cups Superconcentrated Cantonese Chicken Stock (page 256)

⅔ tablespoon Asian light beer, plus additional for flavor

⅓ bunch Chinese watercress

Kosher salt

Sugar

* If you don't have an Asian grocery store near ya, fermented bean curd might be more expensive to buy online. But this is an important ingredient to give the chicken wings and the soup a super umami-savory-licious flavor, so don't skip it!

---

1. Mix wings with fermented bean curd, minced garlic, sugar, and chicken bouillon in a bowl. Cover and marinate overnight.
2. Taste the pineapple, and if it's not sweet enough, toss pineapple rings in a bowl with just enough brown sugar to lightly coat them. (If the pineapple is sweet, skip the brown sugar.) Grill pineapple rings, to bring out the smoky sweetness that money can't buy, for 2 minutes per side, or until you get good grill marks. (You can also sauté in a pan with a little bit of oil if grilling isn't an option for you.) Remove from heat and cut into 1-inch chunks, then set aside in a bowl.
3. Next, sear wings on grill or in pan until the skin looks nice, browned, and food-porn-rific, but do not cook through. Save leftover marinade and set aside.
4. Add wings and leftover marinade to a pot with chicken stock. Bring

to a boil over high heat. Once it starts boiling then lower the heat to a simmer. Cook until wings are tender but not falling off the bone, then add beer and pineapples. Season with salt and sugar and stir.

5. You want a balance of sweet, savory, and not-too-beery. If the soup's too sweet, add a splash of beer. If it's too beery, add a pinch of sugar.

Remove from heat, serve in bowl, garnish with fresh watercress on top, and slurp up the savory soupy goodness that we had to make for our entire family in Orange County for Christmas dinner one year because they were as obsessed with it as I still am.

SALTED PLUM LYCHEE PANNA COTTA

Thi is obsessed with panna cotta—a slightly solid and creamy Italian dessert, not unlike flan, only denser and less bouncy in construction—and her Salted Plum Lychee Panna Cotta is a longstanding staple of our menu, including at Button Mash today. Sweet lychee on the inside, salty plum sauce on the outside, all delicious for our mouths.

BALLS OUT

40–80 SERVINGS

SALTED PLUM SAUCE:

11½ cups water

½ cup salted plum powder

1½ cups lime juice

7 tablespoons agar-agar

PANNA COTTA:

4 tablespoons gelatin powder, or 16½ bronze gelatin sheets/leaves*

3 cups plus 9 cups heavy whipping cream

9 (20-ounce) cans canned lychees or 11¼ pounds fresh lychees, peeled

2 cups milk

2¼ cups sugar

SALTED PLUM SAUCE
(aka fluid gel if you want to get all *Modernist Cuisine* sounding):

1 cup water

2 teaspoons salted plum powder

6⅓ teaspoons lime juice

⅔ teaspoon agar-agar

PANNA COTTA:

1⅓ teaspoons gelatin powder, or 2 bronze gelatin sheets/leaves*

⅓ cup plus 1 cup heavy whipping cream

1 (20-ounce) can lychees or 20 ounces fresh lychees, peeled

3⅔ tablespoons milk

¼ cup sugar

Edible flowers, for garnish (optional)

Pomegranate seeds, for garnish (optional)

* If you have access to these kinds of fancy ingredients from the Internet, gelatin sheets come in bronze, silver, gold, and platinum grade, which signify the "Bloom Strength," or how strong a sheet gels compared to its overall mass.

---

1. **FOR THE SALTED PLUM SAUCE:** Because agar-agar is seaweed-based and fairly delicate to work with, this recipe might be one you can't multitask until you get a good feel for it. Handle with care, and let's hope you don't have to frustratingly do it over and over again.

2. Heat water and salted plum powder in pot over medium heat. When it starts to steam (not boil!), add lime juice and agar-agar. Whisk until agar-agar dissolves. Continue to whisk for 1 minute, or until the mixture thickens. Remove from heat and pour in a container, then let cool to room temperature. Refrigerate to settle. Once it settles, add to a blender and puree until it forms a thicker saucy consistency. Store in fridge until you're ready to bust that bad boy out!

3. **FOR THE PANNA COTTA:** If using gelatin sheets, add to a bowl of ice-cold water and submerge. Soak (aka let the gelatin bloom) for 5–7

minutes, or until the sheets soften. To prevent sheets from breaking down, drain water immediately after the 5–7 minutes and gently wring out remaining water from the sheets, just like you were wringing out a towel.

4. If using powdered gelatin, place gelatin in a bowl and add ⅓ cup heavy cream. Let it sit. Let it bloom.

5. If using a fun mold to shape and pop out your panna cotta, brush a light layer of cooking oil on the bottom and sides.

6. Next, drain syrup from can of lychee (or save for a lychee-flavored cocktail or anything else that could use an "infused" sugary syrup, *yuuuuummers*!). Add lychees to a blender and puree until smooth. Set aside.

7. This next step is very delicate because gelatin in any form is fairly unstable, so this may take some trial and error, based on a balance of your heat and your feel for that heat. You'll know what I mean if you mess up. If you don't, you're a natural-born talent!

8. Heat a pot with milk, sugar, and remaining heavy cream on medium-low heat until sugar dissolves and liquid is warm enough to touch. Like the Salted Plum Sauce, the milk, sugar, and heavy cream should steam but not boil. If you have a thermometer, DO NOT go over 145°F.

9. Next, add gelatin (sheets or powdered in heavy cream), then whisk until gelatin dissolves. This will take a few minutes.

10. Remove from heat, then immediately add lychee puree while the cream is still warm. Mix gently with a spatula.

11. Ladle into ramekins, small bowls, your preferred fancy or not-so-fancy container, or into your pre-oil-brushed mold.

12. Refrigerate, carefully. Gelatin is fairly docile and irritably unstable. As it cools, however, panna cotta should solidify within an hour.

13. If after 2 hours it still hasn't settled, don't fret—you can still recover. Recombine the cream in a pot and warm to right below boiling. Add a tad bit more (bloomed) gelatin, then remove from heat. Repour into molds. Be careful not to add too much gelatin, which will result in a stiff, less creamy panna cotta, more of a superstiff Jell-O than panna cotta.

14. Garnish with a thin layer of Salted Plum Sauce on top of your final plating—do fancy dots or a paintbrush swipe if you would like—and edible flowers (if you somehow got these) and pomegranate seeds (if in season and available). Bon appetit, y'all.

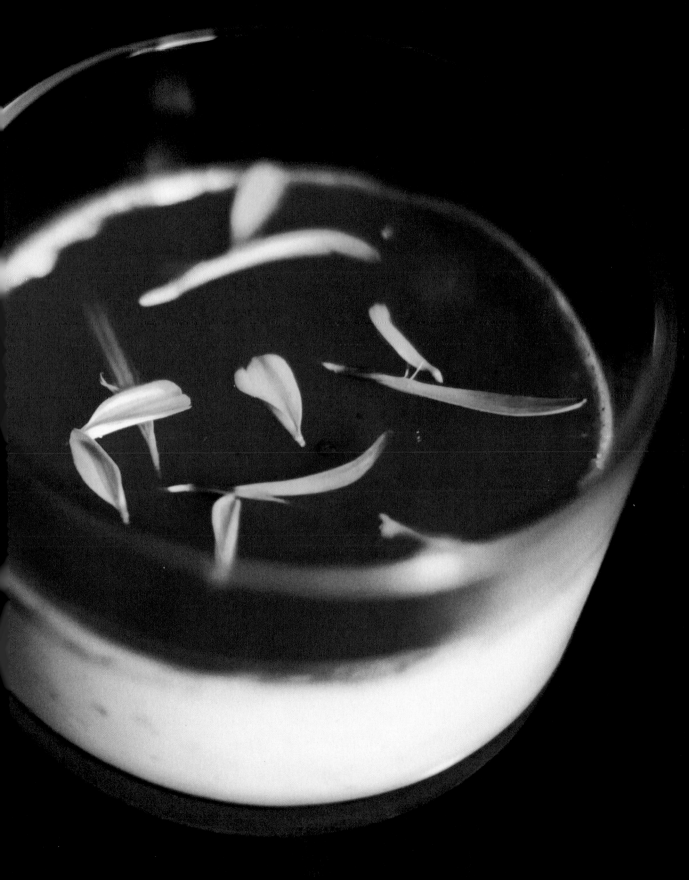

TAIWANESE MINCED PORK W/ PICKLED LICORICE CUCUMBERS

One time Thi made this for me at home, and then I obsessed, begged, pleaded, and finally persuaded her (a recurring theme) to make it for a staff meal back in our lunch days.

It's super comforting and homey—and it gets me a little bit closer to half of Thi's Chinese heritage (she's half Taiwanese/Fukien and another half Cantonese/Hong Kong . . . and she was born in Vietnam . . . if you're keeping track).

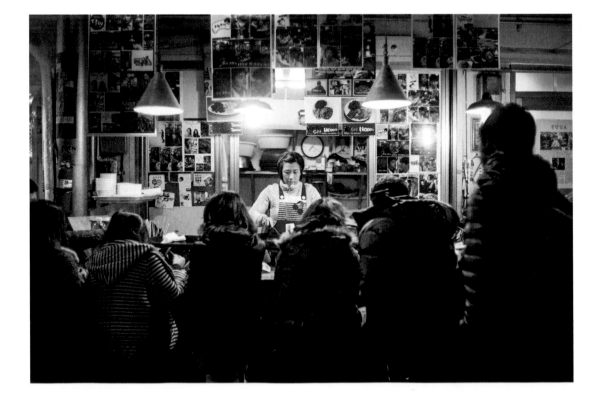

TAIWANESE PICKLED LICORICE CUCUMBERS:

8 Persian cucumbers, washed and patted dry

2 teaspoons distilled white vinegar

10 tablespoons light soy sauce

5 tablespoons sugar

5 tablespoons rice vinegar

4 pieces dried licorice root

MARINADE:

1 pound ground pork

1 tablespoon light soy sauce

2 pinches white pepper

½ tablespoon Chinese cooking wine

1½ teaspoons tapioca starch

SAUCE:

1 tablespoon black vinegar (Koon Chun brand)

½ tablespoon oyster sauce

½ tablespoon soy sauce paste (Ta-Tung brand)

½ tablespoon light soy sauce

½ teaspoon five-spice powder

1 teaspoon sesame oil

¼ cup Taiwanese pickled licorice cucumber liquid

MAIN:

¼ yellow or white onion, finely diced

¼ teaspoon kosher salt

Ground black pepper

1 tablespoon minced garlic

¼ cup diced Taiwanese pickled licorice cucumbers

1½ tablespoons fried garlic

¼ cup plus 2 tablespoons finely chopped scallions

BALLS OUT
40—80 SERVINGS

TAIWANESE PICKLED LICORICE CUCUMBERS:

80 Persian cucumbers, washed and patted dry

6⅔ tablespoons distilled white vinegar

6 cups plus 3 tablespoons light soy sauce

3 cups sugar

3 cups rice vinegar

40 pieces dried licorice root

MARINADE:

20 pounds ground pork

1¼ cups light soy sauce

2½ teaspoons white pepper

10 tablespoons Chinese cooking wine

5 tablespoons tapioca starch (or cornstarch if tapioca starch isn't readily available)

SAUCE:

1¼ cups black vinegar (Koon Chun brand)

10 tablespoons oyster sauce

10 tablespoons soy sauce paste (Ta-Tung brand)

10 tablespoons light soy sauce

10 tablespoons five-spice powder

6⅔ tablespoons sesame oil

5 cups Taiwanese pickled licorice cucumber liquid

MAIN:

5 whole yellow or white onions, finely diced

1⅔ tablespoons kosher salt

Ground black pepper

1¼ cups minced garlic

5 cups diced Taiwanese pickled licorice cucumbers

¾ cup plus 3 tablespoons fried garlic

5 cups plus 2½ cups finely chopped scallions

1. **FOR PICKLED LICORICE CUCUMBERS:** Place whole cucumbers in a bowl and cover with water. Add white vinegar and let sit for 10 minutes. Next, drain liquid, remove cucumbers, cut off ends, and slice into ¼-inch-thick rounds. Combine cut cucumbers, soy sauce, sugar, rice vinegar, and licorice root in a pot and bring to a boil over medium-high heat. Cook for 1 minute, then remove from heat and cool.

2. Transfer to a jar or container. Make sure cucumbers are fully submerged and covered. Refrigerate for at least 24 hours before eating.

3. **FOR MINCED PORKED:** Mix all the marinade ingredients with the pork in a bowl. Set aside and let marinate for 30 minutes.

4. **MIX SAUCE INGREDIENTS:** black vinegar, oyster sauce, soy sauce paste, light soy sauce, five-spice powder, sesame oil, and Taiwanese Pickled Licorice Cucumber liquid in a bowl. Set aside.

5. Heat some cooking oil in a pan on high heat. Once it's hot, add marinated ground pork; flatten out on pan and let cook for 5–7 minutes. Make sure you get a good sear on the pork before turning over, then sear the other side.

6. Start breaking the pork apart in the pan until all the chunks, lumps, and chumps (= chunks + lumps, I'm corny, I know ha-ha) are pretty much gone. (If you are using a nonstick pan, don't use any metal utensils or they will scratch the coating and little bits of it will get in your food!)

7. Lower heat to medium-high and add diced onions. Stir for 1 minute, then add salt, fresh black pepper, and minced garlic. Sauté for 1 more minute.

8. Dice Taiwanese pickled licorice cucumbers, then add, with fried garlic, to pan.

9. Finally, add sauce and scallions; cook and stir for 1 minute.

   Remove from heat, plate over a bed of rice or in a family-style bowl, and garnish with freshly chopped scallions. Oh, Taiwanese comfort food . . . why did it take me so long to discover you and your amazing foods, Taiwan!

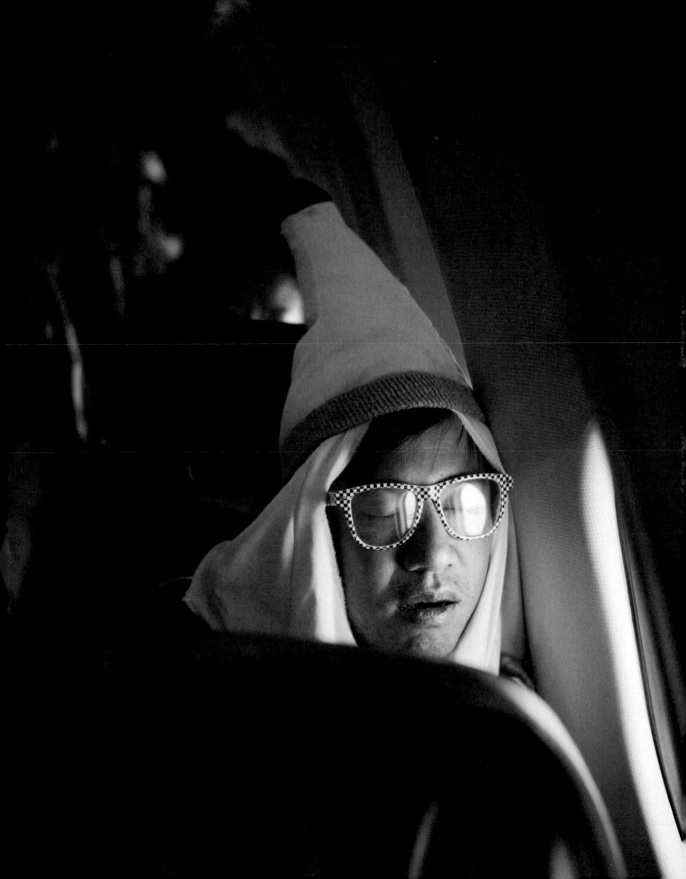

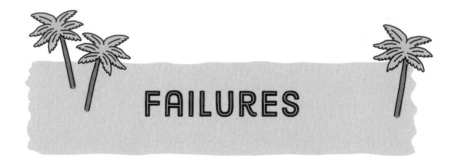

FAILURES

TEN MONTHS AFTER GOING VIRAL, GOING LEGIT, GETTING TONS AND TONS OF PEOPLE LINING UP OUTSIDE OUR RESTAURANT, AND PAYING DOWN OUR CREDIT CARD DEBT, WHICH WE RAN UP IN PURSUIT OF OUR HOPES AND DREAMS, WE WERE TWO MONTHS AWAY FROM GAMING THE SYSTEM, BEATING THE LONG-HELD RULE OF THUMB IN THE RESTAURANT INDUSTRY THAT MOST RESTAURANTS FAIL WITHIN THE FIRST YEAR. AS WE WERE GETTING SO CLOSE TO CROSSING THIS MILESTONE, I WENT BACK AND LOOKED AT ALL THE OTHER RESTAURANTS THAT HAD OPENED AROUND THE SAME TIME WE HAD. THERE WAS ONLY ONE OTHER LEFT, AND ALSO US. TALK ABOUT A DEPRESSINGLY SOBERING REALITY.

There's a Western saying, ". . . then the other shoe dropped," which means to me something is bound to happen eventually, regardless of how hard you try to prevent it. Even with all of the success we were experiencing, our other shoe dropped like ten tons of fucking cinder block bricks—cinder blocks wrapped in the coarsest industrial sandpaper available, constructed and hurled at us to crush our hopes and strip away every remaining layer of pride, dignity . . . and oh yeah, make it hurt so bone deep that I will never forget it. November 2010

was our fateful date. Thinking of this moment in time still brings me to low places every time.

We knew nothing about running a restaurant. The previous owners hadn't known much either, but we learned from them—the blind leading the blind. Banana suits and lederhosen were part of the extreme measures I used to promote the place. LA legend Laurent Quenioux cooked some amazing meals with us, including some marijuana dinners that got my ugly mug in the *LA Times* and I'm sure on the DEA's watch list. None of it made sense, but

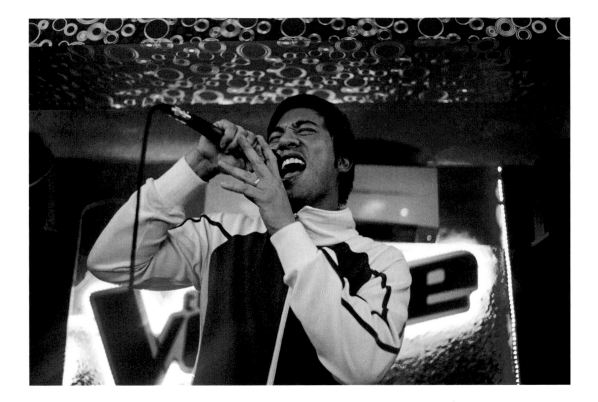

it worked, and Starry Kitchen got coverage in places like the *New York Times*.

Simple tough-love fact about myself: I'm not great at being a responsible person! I ignored bills that weren't immediate to focus on the big picture, pushing them off as I was steering the crazy manic momentum we had because I was DETERMINED to beat that one-year statistic—and if we failed, none of those bills would matter anyway.

What I wasn't taking into account (literally) was SALES TAX. In the State of California, contrary to my naïve assumption (and what I still think defies common sense), sales tax is not reported by your cash register/electronic point-of-sale system. We, the business, have to collect

that money, hold on to it for almost three months, and when the time comes around, we are trusted to honestly report it and pay the piper what is due.

When business is slow and that business might not be able to afford payroll? Do you think the staff would accept, "Ya know, it's been a slow month so I can't make payroll, and I have this money I owe the government about two months from now but I can't simply hand that over to you to pay your bills, feed your family, stay afloat because, well, you guys get it, right? BECAUSE GOVERNMENT!"

No, that conversation doesn't happen. It's not the employees' problem or responsibility to know about or deal with any of that.

What does all this amount to? The Board of Equalization, my most beloved organization (insert heavy sarcasm HERE) within the State of California, sends me letters informing me that I'm delinquent. I realize the error of my ways, report my sales (honestly), and then go on my merry daily way of keeping the Starry Kitchen train going. I then get a "friendly" call from a collector at the Board of Equalization, during which she basically demands ALL the money I owe for nearly three quarters' (nine months) worth of uncollected taxes immediately, right then, and definitely right there.

I go silent for a moment. I think about how much I reported, how much I owe my staff in payroll coming up and being the pragmatic negotiator, I believe I can work my way out of anything as long as we just talk it through, "Oh, I'm sorry, I just don't have that kind of cash at the moment but I'd love to figure out a deal with you and pay some now and the rest later." She then curtly responds, "No, we can't do that. We have to have it all, or we'll have to take action."

She doesn't budge. I thought she might be amenable to talking more because the State of California can't be a petty gangster (can they?) and wants small businesses to flourish and grow to last for years to come, right?

Simple answer: NOPE. The State of California *is* a gangster, they're broke, and your problems are not their problems. End of conversation.

Two weeks after that tantalizing conversation, I was filling my car up with gas . . . and my debit card was declined, which was odd because I knew we had $12,000 in the bank. My heart plummeted so low and hard that

I'm pretty sure it was sighted somewhere on the other side of the world, somewhere in the Eastern Hemisphere as a pitifully shrunken heart that looked like it might have belonged to a small animal that had died long ago.

After many phone calls with my bank I figured it out: The Tony Soprano of governmental agencies (yes, YOU, Board of Equalization) had done the unfathomable. They had levied (aka taken) ALL my money, which was now their money, with complete disregard for our staff, our business, our well-being, our ability to grow as a business, our *anything* because, hey, it's *theirs,* and who gives a fuck what happens to us, the people we employ, and the financial ecosystem we contribute to?

After this, Thi wanted to shut down for good. This was absolutely the worst thing that could happen to us. (But in fact, ah-ha, the blows of all-time-lows didn't stop coming and DID get worse . . . I tear up and want to get into a fetal position just thinking about all the mind-numbing pain sometimes—it still hurts.)

And to that point, the next immediate worst thing that had to happen (because "when it rains . . . you drown") was preparing to have a conversation with our staff about their payroll the NEXT FUCKING DAY!

There was only one way to handle this: Be brutally honest and tell the staff this ludicrous story, hope they believed me, and hope they didn't walk right out the door. I still remember the glazed looks on the faces of my predominantly Hispanic staff members as I told them, "Hey, I don't have your money. The State of California took it, and I can't make payroll." I doubt there was much of a language barrier when it came to that conversation, even if I personally wanted one to exist just to cushion the blow to my personal pride so I could think to myself, "Oh, maybe they didn't understand all of it so they won't completely hate me." But they *did* understand, and they *did* hate me. I can't blame them. I really looked like a shitty boss at the time. Fortunately, I was able to pay them out of the restaurant's daily sales until I could pay them in full, though I was late with their paychecks for the next three months because of the levy from the Board of Equalization.

But that wasn't even the end of it. Three months later, at the beginning of lunch service, after months of trying to get caught up in pay, my sanity, and life in general, I bitched at the kitchen staff (being the boss) about an issue I had bitched at them about multiple times before. This is when the proverbial straw broke the proverbial camel's back. One of the cooks retaliated and asked about their money, which wasn't supposed to be relevant here, but all's fair in love and the kitchen, right? I didn't want to answer him, partially because I wanted to get through the lunch shift and partially because I was caught off guard and didn't have a good answer. When I didn't answer, that cook left. Then another cook left. The three other cooks stayed to help us get through the shift, but they left after service. They ALL left. We were not just royally fucked but COMPLETELY and TOTALLY fucked. Could our ride, rise, and continual rollercoaster over one year shut us down as quickly as that?

Morale (and staff) was low, so I really had no other option than to close shop that night and decided to take everyone left out to eat and get drunk. ("Celebrating our failure!") We all rode out to Dan Sung Sa, one of the oldest pub food restaurants in Koreatown, where we proceeded to get wasted. I also invited along some friends to revel in our misfortune. We talked, drank lots of mixed *soju* (a Korean alcohol that can really fuck you—at least me—up, made with ethanol but masked by a fruity or milk flavor), and ate a ton of chicken wings and gizzards and all sorts of food I don't remember ordering.

And then our friends hit me with the least obvious Starry Kitchen–like solution: our unemployed friends who ain't got shit to do could lend a hand!

These friends would help what was left of our staff—and help out they did. They were REALLY good, honestly better than some of the much more seasoned staff for a very simple reason: They CARED. And *caring* is so much more important than people think. More important than skill, in many cases, and why I now value loyalty over skill. Sure, experience means a lot, but when someone *cares* for the people running an establishment, for the food they are making and serving to others, and for what people think of their work, and/or they believe that the work they're doing is worth their time and energy— hot DAAAAAAAAAAAAMN, they can be GREAT! Amazing! . . . and what a fucking great lesson (oh yeah, we also survived ☺).

The thing I learned most from this first of many (ofttimes hilarious) shitty experiences is that it really wasn't that unique. This situation would resurface in many different incarnations, with many other "white devil" culprits that I would love to blame, and would continually be part of our narrative.

4½ CHEESE BACON MAC AND CHEESE

We have a few random dishes with some pretty random explanations for why we make them . . . and I honestly don't have a good explanation for why we have Mac and Cheese, but I can tell you that Thi LOVES to stir-fry with macaroni pasta. And a former Michelin star chef, who staged with us in 2011, introduced the roux into this recipe and made our Mac and Cheese better (end of story).

2–4 SERVINGS

4 cups whole milk plus additional for reheating

1 cup manufacturing cream or heavy (whipping) cream *

0.625 ounces lemongrass stalk, smashed †

0.75 ounces ginger, crushed

1 ounce Thai chili, cut lengthwise, with seeds

4.12 ounces unsalted butter

½ cup flour

2.5 ounces parmesan cheese, shredded

5.5 ounces mild cheddar cheese, diced very small

4.375 ounces Velveeta, diced very small

4.75 ounces gruyère cheese, diced very small

7 ounces Monterey jack cheese, diced very small

¼ teaspoon ground white pepper

1 teaspoon kosher salt

Elbow macaroni, cooked

Caramelized onions

Fried shallots

Bacon, cooked and crispy ‡

Freshly cracked black pepper

* Manufacturing cream is not the same as heavy whipping cream; it has a higher butterfat content and tends to be smoother, but it is not as readily available as its whipping cream cousin.

† This recipe depends on mass/weight more than others, hence the precise measurements. The ratio of cheeses took us a long time to nail down, and we needed more precision to achieve the texture and balance that we were happy with. We hope you appreciate the fruits (and cheeses) of our hard work (and don't mind all the dated imperial system measurements)!

‡ The PRO decadent move is save all that bacon fat, and replace the butter in the recipe with it to make a bacon blond roux.

BALLS OUT
40–80 SERVINGS

10 quarts whole milk plus additional for reheating

10 cups manufacturing cream or heavy (whipping) cream *

6.25 ounces lemongrass stalk, smashed †

7½ ounces ginger, crushed

10 ounces Thai chili, cut lengthwise, with seeds

2.57 pounds unsalted butter

5 cups flour

1.56 pounds parmesan cheese, shredded

3.43 pounds mild cheddar cheese, diced very small

2.73 pounds Velveeta, diced very small

2.96 pounds gruyère cheese, diced very small

4.37 pounds Monterey jack cheese, diced very small

2½ teaspoons ground white pepper

3⅓ tablespoons kosher salt

1. Heat milk, cream, lemongrass, ginger, and Thai chilies in a pan under medium-low heat. Once the milk starts to steam, remove from heat and allow the flavors to infuse for 5–10 minutes. Afterwards, strain and dispose of chilies, ginger, and lemongrass.

2. Be prepared to stay at the stove for the next step because we're making a roux. If you need to step away for any reason, remove roux from heat.

3. In a pot on medium heat, add butter. Once butter is melted, start making a blond roux by slowly adding in flour and constantly mixing or whisking the flour into the butter, keeping the consistency smooth. Do this until all the flour has been incorporated.

4. Continue mixing for about 5 minutes until the roux turns a milky yellow blond color. Now strain the infused milk through a chinois or fine sieve into the roux, mixing out any lumps constantly. Make sure it's all smooth.

5. Next, add in cheeses one at a time, stirring constantly until each cheese is completely melted (we haven't found the order for adding the cheeses to make a huge difference, til y'all prove us wrong). The smaller the dice, the faster the cheese will melt.

6. Add white pepper and salt.

7. When the cheese is fully incorporated, remove from heat. (Note: It may have a slightly granular consistency because of the gruyère, but gruyère is too good to not include!) Strain the cheese through a chinois into another pot. The main thing to know about using a chinois is to force the liquid through the fine mesh using a wooden spoon or spatula (otherwise, you're going to be there a LONG time waiting for that cheese to pass through).

8. The hardest part is now done. It's ready to be served immediately. If being served at a later time, however, keep the cheese warm and runny by holding it over a double boiler (aka *bain-marie*), which is quite simple. You'll need two pots, one of which can comfortably sit on top of the other. One will hold water on medium heat, while the other pot will just rest on top. This will ensure that the cheese doesn't burn, and it will maintain the consistency as well.

9. If you want to use the cheese at a later date, let cool to room temperature, cover, and refrigerate. Reheat using the double-boiler technique.

10. If the cheese becomes too thick, add a little more milk to thin it out.

Serve over a bowl of elbow macaroni and top with caramelized onions, fried shallots, crispy bacon bits, and a quick twist of freshly cracked black pepper—just like we used to serve it at our lunch spot back in yesteryear. MERCI! Or if you're from Texas like us, serve it with super thin flour tortilla chips, dip 'em, and get your chips and queso ON! (Maybe add some Rotel for good chips and queso measure if you go that route.)

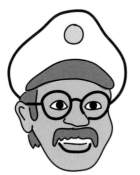

VIETNAMESE EGGROLLS (AKA CHA GIO)

I've said it before, I still say it a lot, and I know my friends from other Asian ethnicities may hate me for saying this, but I've tried about every ethnic eggroll I've been able to find, and I still contend that Vietnamese eggrolls are the best, if not the most complicated, of all eggrolls.

2–4 SERVINGS

½ pound shrimp, peeled and deveined (see The SK Way, page 144)

1 pound ground pork

½ cup dried wood ear mushrooms, soaked in hot water and softened

1 cup shredded carrots

1 cup shredded taro root

½ small onion, finely diced

4 teaspoons minced garlic

1 tablespoon minced shallots

1 teaspoon kosher salt

2 teaspoons ground black pepper

1 package eggroll wrappers

½ bundle dried bean thread noodles, soaked in hot water, softened and cut in half

1 tablespoon sugar

1 tablespoon fish sauce

1 teaspoon chicken bouillon

1 large egg plus more, just in case

Green or red leaf lettuce, leaves individually cleaned and stacked

Vermicelli, cooked

Pickled Shredded Carrots and Daikon (page 250)

Mint or *tiato*, or both, cleaned and stemmed

Cilantro, thoroughly cleaned

Coco Rico Vietnamese Fish Sauce (page 240)

BALLS OUT
40–80 SERVINGS

5 pounds shrimp, peeled and deveined

10 pounds ground pork

5 cups dried wood ear mushrooms, soaked in hot water and softened

10 cups shredded carrots

10 cups shredded taro root

5 small onions, finely diced

13⅓ tablespoons minced garlic

10 tablespoons minced shallots

3⅓ tablespoons kosher salt

6⅔ tablespoons ground black pepper

10 packages eggroll wrappers

5 bundles dried bean thread noodles, soaked in hot water, softened and cut in half

10 tablespoons sugar

10 tablespoons fish sauce

3⅓ tablespoons chicken bouillon

10 large eggs plus more, just in case

1. In a food processor, blend the shrimp into a paste-like consistency. Don't puree it, or you'll ruin it ("Oh NO!"). Add pork, then blend to combine. If your food processor isn't large enough to blend both together, blend them separately and then transfer to a bowl and hand mix thoroughly.

2. Transfer the pork-shrimp mixture to a bowl (if it isn't in one already), then add mushrooms, carrots, taro root, onion, garlic, shallots, salt, and pepper. Mix. To test the seasoning, sauté a tiny patty of meat in a pan on high heat with a little bit of oil and cook it all the way through. Taste it and adjust seasoning as needed.

3. Next, beat egg in a separate bowl. Set egg wash aside.

4. Open eggroll wrappers. Cover exposed wrappers with a damp (not dripping wet) towel to keep them moist while wrapping; they will dry out quickly if you don't do this.

5. Take a single wrapper and lay it in front of you like a diamond. Place 1 tablespoon eggroll filling onto the wrapper, not quite in the middle, just a tad bit closer to your body. Next, spread filling from left to right, just a tad short of both edges.

6. With a spoon or the tip of your fingers, dampen the top corner of the diamond with a bit of egg wash so that the wrapper will stick and stay together when rolling.

7. Fold in the left and right corners. Next, fold the point nearest you in and roll (while pinching in the sides) toward the opposite (top) corner.

8. Line a baking sheet with parchment paper and place eggrolls on it as you finish rolling. Cover finished egg rolls with another damp towel to prevent them from drying out and unraveling.

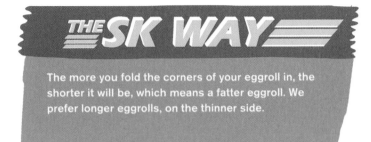

THE SK WAY

The more you fold the corners of your eggroll in, the shorter it will be, which means a fatter eggroll. We prefer longer eggrolls, on the thinner side.

9. Heat 2 inches of oil in a pot over medium-high heat until it reaches 350°F. Fry eggrolls for 6–8 minutes, turning frequently, until the skins turn golden and crunchy. (Rolls should bubble when they touch the oil. If they don't bubble, the oil isn't hot enough.) Remove eggrolls, shake off excess oil, and drip dry on a plate lined with paper towels. Let cool for 5 minutes.

10. Serve stacked Lincoln Log–style with sides of lettuce, vermicelli, Pickled Shredded Carrots and Daikon, mint, cilantro, and a side of Coco Rico Vietnamese Fish Sauce.

If you want advice on how to eat all of that (as I've seen how unobvious it is to people at Button Mash, and I say that sincerely): First off, remember that "less is more" and place a little bit of vermicelli in a piece of lettuce large enough to wrap up an eggroll, some Pickled Carrots and Daikon, one to two mint leaves, one cilantro stem with leaves on, and one eggroll; wrap it all up, dip it in the fish sauce, and really . . . REALLY make sweet love to your mouth with all the flavors and textures of the most complex eggroll known to humankind!

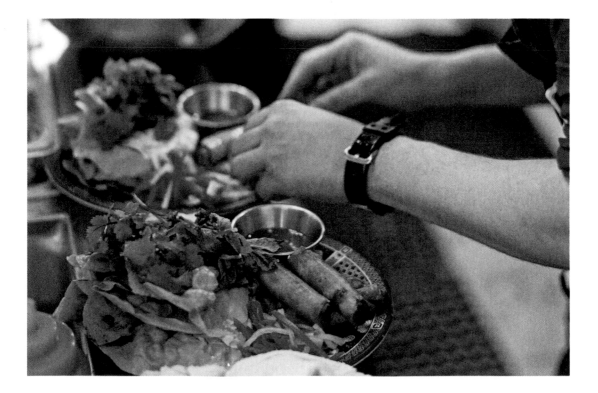

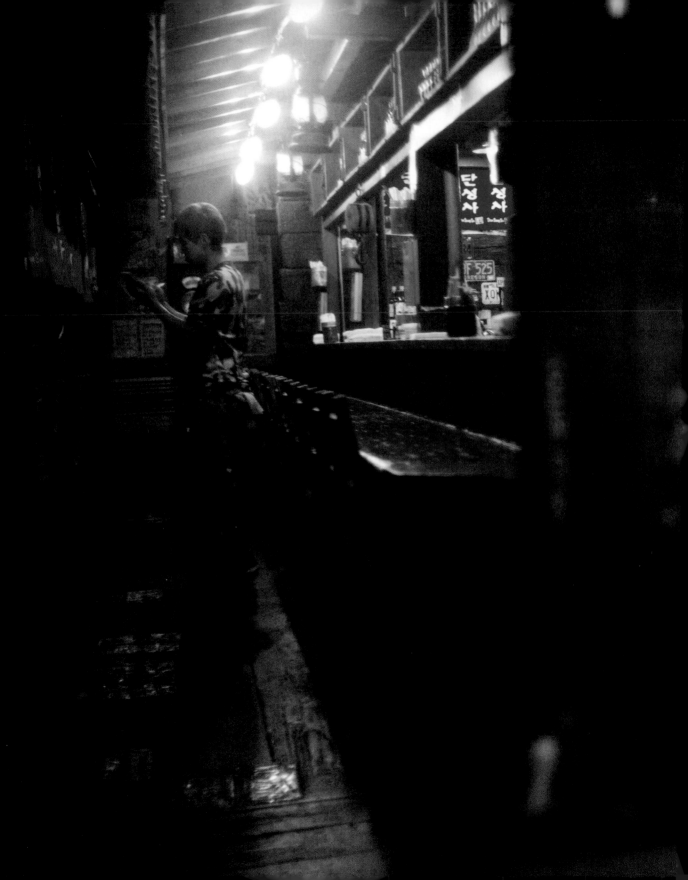

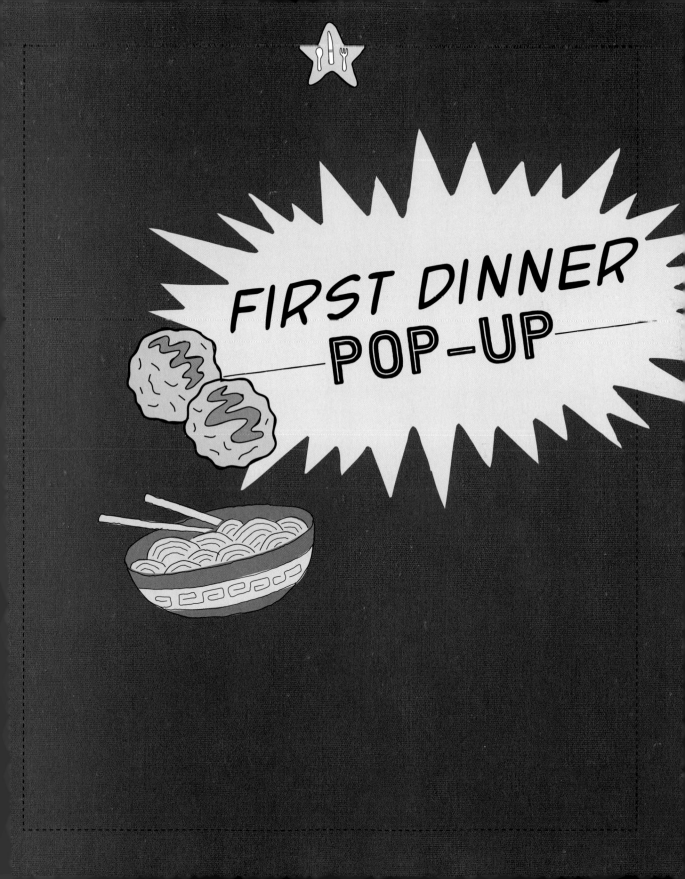

FIRST DINNER POP-UP

BANANA SUIT CONFIDENTIAL

MY BELOVED BANANA SUIT IS THE OUTFIT OF ALL (15+) OUTFITS. FOR BETTER OR FOR WORSE, **I AM MOST SYNONYMOUS WITH THE SUIT.** I WILLED THAT SUIT AND STARRY KITCHEN INTO EXISTENCE, THOUGH I'VE ACTUALLY WORN OUT FOUR SUITS OVER THE YEARS.

If I were ever to include FAQs on our website, I would definitely add the following frequently-asked-at-every-turn questions about my banana suit:

So, why the banana suit?
Because I'm the owner of Starry Kitchen and because I can. (Subtext: I *am* HR, BITCH!)

So, are bananas featured in your food?
Not really.

So, why the banana suit again?
Oh, you want to know the backstory. Gotcha and got it. Well . . .

I'll be honest—the banana suit, to me, is just a yellow piece of cloth I slide on with some pretty cool accessories and go to TOWN with. But MAN, for most other people, it's absolute CRAZINESS. And I do get a whole lot CRAZIER when I'm in it, so that would make sense. For me, "thinking outside the box" is easy because I believe "the box" is far smaller than people think. And stepping outside the imaginary mime-like walls doesn't have to be a BIG step if your toe is already outside the box. Once you're out, you're out. I do believe in breaking those barriers, and the best part of the banana suit is that it gives people permission to step out of their comfort zones a little. If they do that, they become a little more comfortable in their skin and, as a result, are more likely to do something slightly crazy, or at least a little crazier than they'd normally contemplate.

When that happens, as far as I'm concerned, I've done my job.

I started wearing the banana suit when I was working on my final indie film, *White on Rice*, a charming romantic comedy about a misguided Japanese man-child who finds himself through his extended family in the United States and falls in love with a girl (get ready for it) . . . IN A BANANA SUIT. (Said Banana-Suit-Girl was played by my friend Joy Osmanski, who you'll see on TV sometimes!) I really love this film. If you haven't seen it, Netflix that shit, bitches! The film was screened at the Asian American Film Festival here in Los Angeles, and I just happened to be one of the festival judges. After watching the film, I was so floored by how much the audience loved it and how heartwarming it was that I totally crossed the festival judging line (sanctioned by: no one) and told the filmmaker, Dave Boyle, that I wanted to help him find distribution for his film or release it myself, because THAT was actually my job at the time.

Dave and I started working together to release and promote the film ourselves, well outside the studio system. To promote the film, we set up a grassroots marketing and publicity campaign. Out of the blue, but definitely inspired by the character in the film, I asked Dave to let me borrow the banana suit. When he asked me why, I wasn't sure, but I thought I might be able to work some magic in it.

The first time I wore the banana suit, I crashed a parade in Little Tokyo with a string of very nervous volunteers and found out that the No. 1 request for the life of the banana suit would be to have me do the "Peanut Butter Jelly Time" dance more times than it's ever been performed in the history of humankind

since that was the hottest thing banana suits were associated with at the time . . . and oh yeah, because it's FUCKING HILARIOUS! ☺

And then I figured out, WOW, banana suits really make people smile and laugh and let go. It's the least creepy outfit to attract both males and females, both young and old. It's like a magnet. It's "It's a Small World After All" magical. I couldn't believe it. That's why I wear the banana suit today.

The tail end of the *White on Rice* release happened to time perfectly with the rise and sudden explosion of our illegal+underground restaurant that would take Starry Kitchen out of our apartment into legitimacy. After we went legit, I VOWED I would use the banana suit only for good, because as Uncle Ben told Peter Parker, "with great power comes great responsibility." I should stress here that practicing patience and restraint is not at all like me. But I waited a long and arduous five months until I finally broke out the suit again. This was July 2010, when my good friend Shawna Dawson, LA hospitality marketing impresario, invited Starry Kitchen to join her crazy explosive LA Street Food Fest at the Rose Bowl (and this was the LAST time we were able to serve on the extremely magical Rose Bowl field, too—oh man, it's pretty! I ran across it with security chasing me in my banana suit, and rolled around on it a lot, too!). I don't think she knew what she was in for when I told her I'd bring my banana suit out for her, and actually . . . even with the *White on Rice* experience, I didn't know what I was in for either.

That fateful day is also the day I came up with the Crispy Tofu Balls catchphrase: "Please enjoy our balls in your mouth." For its premiere, I asked our good friends to make a sign. If you remember

July 2010, this was back when the social media app Foursquare was still . . . JUST Foursquare. All of my savvy friends approached the LA Street Food Fest with one main purpose: to create a MEGA swarm of about 250+ people checking into the same location, which in the early days of social media was an impressive number of people.

The energy before the gates opened was frantic, palpable, and downright nerve-racking.

We were trying to set up the booth and get organized, all while our friends, the true heroes of that day, were busy slaving away frying our tofu balls in the dark, barely lit crevices of the Rose Bowl tunnels, because I thought I could save money by using tiny tabletop propane burners to fry HUGE pots of balls—not the last time my cheap ambition nearly did us in. When the gates were about to open, I put on my banana

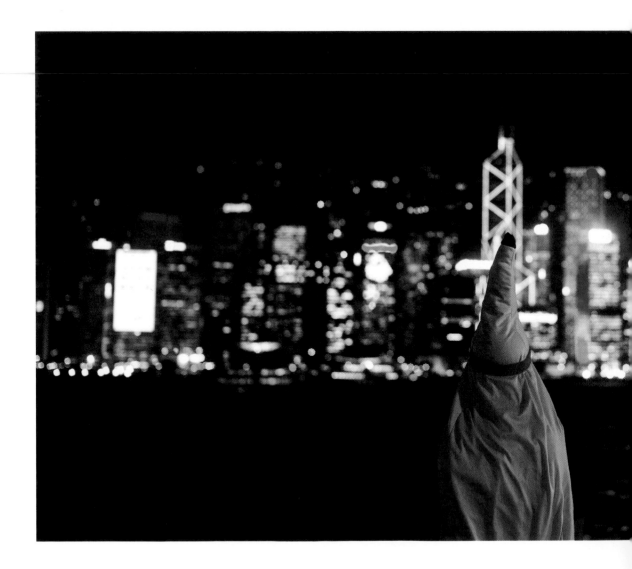

suit as if I were getting ready for battle. Then I slipped on my now superinfamous sandwich board like I'm a six-pack-sporting Spartan in armor from *300* because "THIS. IS. STARRY KITCHEEEEEEEN."

Since we've now done tons of these events, I can tell you that people normally spread out to find whatever type of food catches their eye, or they go straight to the hottest ticket at the

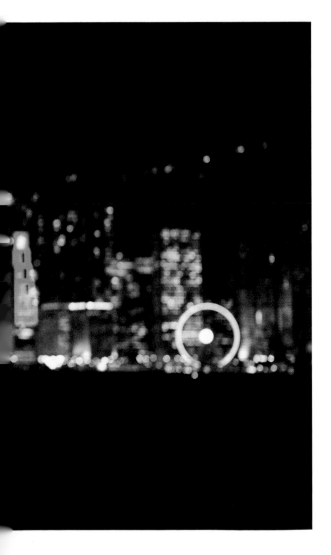

place. Believe me, we were neither the hottest ticket nor were tofu balls in high demand. And yet, when those gates opened, EVERYONE made a bee-line for us. Even today I'm still not quite sure why, but as the horde of humanity neared the Starry Kitchen booth, I'm pretty sure they were coming because of my banana suit. The onslaught of people, jokes, pictures, social media posts, TV interviews, even You-Tube celebrities like Smosh continued through-out the afternoon. And everyone blew us up even more by sharing our elusive underground story. I welcomed the attention for Starry Kitchen, and I realized that the banana suit was now the restaurant's mascot, its unofficial thing, even though it had nothing do with our illegal or legit undertaking until that moment.

Since then, I've introduced probably twenty different outfits, including lederhosen, a huge Spanish sombrero, Darth Vader, an inflatable tauntaun (watch *The Empire Strikes Back* if you haven't, and then you'll know the amazingness of having your own inflatable tauntaun, where your legs are the legs of the animal and there are teeny lil' legs above for your superdeformed body . . . HA-HA-HA), super-short-shorts '80s guy with matching Drakkar Noir cologne to match ("Smell like the '80s, pick up ladies . . . like the '80s!"). Whenever I wear one of those costumes instead of the banana suit, without fail, people always ask, "WHERE'S THE BANANA SUIT!?"

And just like that, I became that one-hit wonder, the Gloria Gaynor of the LA food scene, and people only ever want one thing. And you know what? I pretty much do give it to the fans almost every single time because . . . I *DO* love wearing my banana suit!

CITRUS SESAME TOFU

We're not necessarily known for our refreshing dishes, so this one might seem like it comes out of left field. It's really refreshing. And . . . so . . . GOOD! Such a great palate cleanser and . . . it looks fancy—fancy enough to impress your (and our) bougie friends.

2–4 SERVINGS

BALLS OUT
40–80 SERVINGS

10 (11-ounce) tubes silken tofu, cut widthwise into ¾-inch-thick discs[†]

2½ teaspoons kosher salt

3⅓ tablespoons sugar

2½ ounces ginger

10 tablespoons rice vinegar

10 tablespoons vegetable oil

3¾ ounces Korean sesame leaves, stemmed[*]

2 cups freshly squeezed orange juice

⅛ ounce orange zest plus additional for topping

---

1 (11-ounce) tube silken tofu, cut widthwise into ¾-inch-thick discs[*]

¼ teaspoon kosher salt

1 teaspoon sugar

¼ ounce ginger

1 tablespoon rice vinegar

1 tablespoon vegetable oil

⅓ ounce Korean sesame leaves, stemmed[†]

3¼ tablespoons orange juice

Whole Korean sesame leaves, for plating

Pinch of orange zest plus additional for topping

Fresh ground black pepper, for garnish

[*] Silken tofu in a tube might be hard for some of y'all to find locally because it's more specialized; even some Asian markets don't have it. If you can't find it, any silken or extra soft tofu will work, but it's important to get it extra soft (and extra sexy).

[†] Easiest to find in Korean grocery stores, some Asian grocery stores will carry these too. The best is when they're as large as a human hand, fragrant, and can almost stand straight on their own.

1. Set tofu aside and combine all other ingredients in a blender to make sauce.
2. Blend away, and taste the sauce. It should be lightly sweet, just a tad savory, with a little bit of bright citrusy flavor. Very light, not too strong.
3. Cover and let sit for 15 minutes (though refrigerating overnight is always best).
4. When you're ready to eat, lay a whole sesame leaf on a small plate and top with a slice of tofu. Have fun with it. Mix sauce and top tofu with a tablespoonful, or just enough to cover tofu slice.
5. Garnish with a pinch of orange zest and a sprinkle of freshly cracked black pepper.

   Bon appétit! . . . or something similarly French. Tres bien! Oui, OUI!☺

BÓ LÁ LỐT [GRILLED BEEF WRAPPED IN SESAME LEAVES]

Bò bảy món (aka seven courses of beef) is one of the greatest Vietnamese culinary delights most people have never heard of. The Starry Kitchen version of one (of the seven courses) differs from the traditional dish. Most recipes use the uniquely sharp and Southeast Asian betel leaf, but we use sesame leaves, because . . . well, after eating a shit ton of Korean food in K-town, we grew to love Korean sesame leaves like they were our own, or at least our tasty adopted child of a culture we would love to call our own. K-town (eating and karaoke/noraebang) FOREVER!

BALLS OUT
40–80 SERVINGS

160 whole large Korean sesame leaves, stemmed

AROMATICS:

6⅔ tablespoons finely minced shallots

¾ cup minced garlic

2½ cups finely minced lemongrass

MEAT:

10 pounds 80–20 ground chuck

1 cup plus 2 tablespoons fish sauce

4⅓ tablespoons five-spice powder

4⅓ tablespoons palm (aka coconut) sugar*

2 tablespoons turmeric powder

2–4 SERVINGS

16 whole large Korean sesame leaves, stemmed

AROMATICS:

⅔ tablespoon finely minced shallots

1⅓ tablespoons minced garlic

¼ cup finely minced lemongrass

MEAT:

1 pound 80–20 ground chuck

5⅔ teaspoons fish sauce

1¼ teaspoons five-spice powder

1⅓ palm (aka coconut) sugar*

⅔ teaspoon turmeric powder

6-inch bamboo skewers, presoaked in water overnight

Cooking oil, for brushing

GARNISHES:

White or black sesame seeds

Red bell pepper, finely diced

Pickled Shredded Carrots and Daikon (page 250) on the side

* If the palm sugar is the clumpy kind, blend it in a food processor until it's a near-fine grain.

---

1. Bring a pot of lightly salted water to boil over high heat. In a bowl large enough to soak sesame leaves, prepare an ice water bath.
2. Once the water is boiling, oil leaves for 5 seconds, then remove and immediately submerge in ice water bath. Remove leaves, shake off excess water, pat each leaf dry, then drip dry on a bed of paper towels. Because you're going to use the leaves to wrap the beef, make sure to keep them as whole as possible.

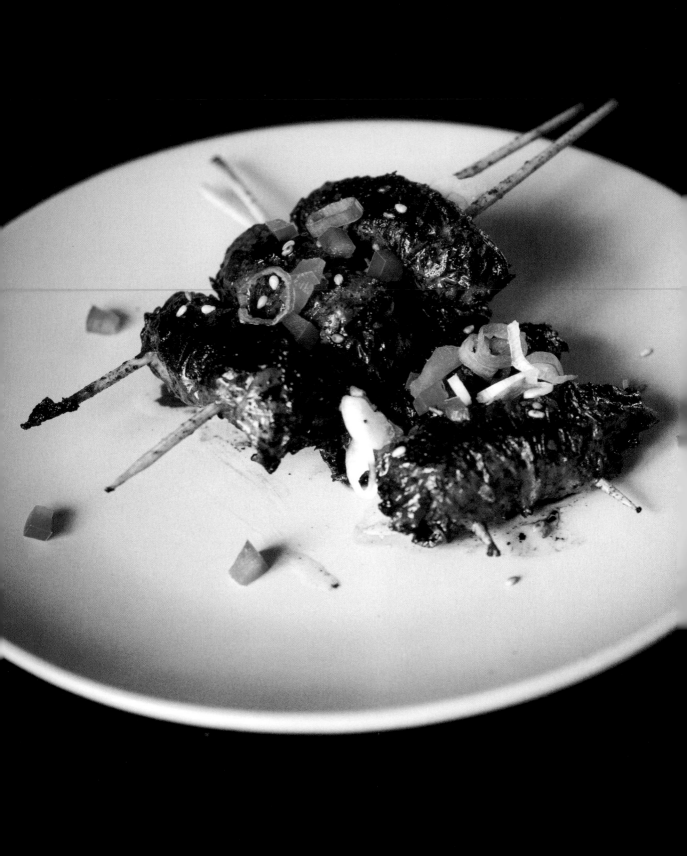

3. Heat wok/pan with a dash of cooking oil over medium-high heat. Sauté shallots for 3 minutes, or until they become translucent. Remove pan from heat, and immediately stir in garlic and lemongrass. Set aside and let cool to room temperature.

4. In the meantime, combine beef, fish sauce, five-spice powder, palm sugar, and turmeric in bowl. Add cooled-down sautéed aromatics (shallots, garlic, lemongrass) and mix.

5. One by one, lay out blanched sesame leaves, shiny-side up, with the top of the leaf pointing away from you. Drop a tablespoon of meat in the lower middle end of the leaf and form a small log widthwise across the stem, then fold in the sides and slowly roll up until closed. Lay flat on a tray and repeat until you're out of beef or sesame leaves, whichever comes first.

6. Next, skewer as many "logs" with two skewers (or toothpicks), keeping about 1 inch between the parallel skewers. Brush wrapped logs o' beef with oil. Repeat until all wrapped beef is skewered and oil-brushed.

7. If you have a grill, place directly on a rack over a medium-high flame. Cook for 3 minutes per side, or until the leaves are slightly charred.

8. If you don't have a grill, sauté in a pan over medium-high heat with some cooking oil. Make sure the pan is hot before adding the skewers—and keep the skewers in place, or the leaves will unravel as they cook.

Stack skewers on top of one another in a crisscross pattern. Garnish with sesame seeds and red bell peppers, and serve with a side of pickles to balance out the flavors.

VIETNAMESE BEEF CARPACCIO

Thin slices o' tender raw beef . . . soaked in the flavors of my peoples of Vietnam and Southeast Asia . . . I think that's about all the talk we need on this one . . . Good talk!

BALLS OUT
40–80 SERVINGS

5 cups lemon juice

5 cups lime juice

1½ cups sugar

10 pounds (8-ounce) ribeye beef, thinly sliced

1¼ cups Coco Rico Vietnamese Fish Sauce (page 240)

5 red onions, thinly sliced

5 yellow onions, thinly sliced

1¼ cups roasted peanuts, coarsely chopped, for garnish

1¼ cups fried shallots, for garnish

10 Fresno chilies, finely sliced widthwise, for garnish

2–4 SERVINGS

¼ cup lemon juice

¼ cup lime juice

1¼ tablespoons sugar

1 (8-ounce) ribeye beef, thinly sliced

1 tablespoon Coco Rico Vietnamese Fish Sauce (page 240)

¼ red onion, thinly sliced

¼ yellow onion, thinly sliced

1 tablespoon roasted peanuts, coarsely chopped, for garnish

Mint chiffonade, for garnish

Basil chiffonade, for garnish

1 tablespoon fried shallots, for garnish

½ Fresno chili pepper, finely sliced widthwise, for garnish

1. Combine lemon juice, lime juice, and sugar in a bowl. Mix until sugar dissolves.
2. Pound each slice of beef flat on a cutting board or flat surface. Next, submerge beef into the lemon-lime mix bowl. *Sploosh.* Cover and refrigerate for 2–3 hours. (After the first hour, stir to prevent the sugar from settling.)
3. When ready to eat, remove beef slices individually and gently wring out lemon-lime mix. Lay flat on a plate and pour on just enough of the smooth stylin's of Coco Rico Vietnamese Fish Sauce to cover the beef.

    Garnish with red and yellow onions, peanuts, mint, basil, fried shallots, and Fresno chilies. Presto! You gots yourself a fancy and delectable appetizer (or a really good cold-cut Banh Mi sammie—I just came up with that and am going to try it out right now!).

THE SK WAY

A note about the ribeye. When I say "thinly sliced," I mean prosciutto-almost-paper-thin thinly sliced. There are three ways to go about this, "buddy":

1. Go to any Asian grocery store or any store that happens to have a shabu-shabu section—Japanese for hot pot. *Mmmmmm, MMMMMM.* They're sure to have presliced meats ready to go. "Yatta!"—Chun-Li, *Street Fighter 2.*
2. Go to a butcher counter and—politely—ask the butcher to slice the ribeye for you.
3. You COULD do it yourself, but it requires a steady hand and very sharp knife. We used to slice the ribeye by hand at our Fashion District pop-up, but I wouldn't recommend it. (We were also cutting large slabs of ribeye, which are far easier to slice than a steak.) If all you have is a steak, I wouldn't recommend trying to slice it as it is a recipe to get hurt. If you ignore this warning, here's a pro tip: Stick the steak in the freezer before cutting. Don't freeze it all the way though—just enough to harden it so you can hold onto it and cut through it.

GREEN CURRY SILKY TOFU

This dish is a spicy-ass green curry blend, married with unlikely sexy-silky-smooth fried tofu, lightly crispy on the outside but wonderfully soft on the inside. Served with Okinawan sweet potatoes . . . so SO savory and so much fun varying textures in your mouth . . . I LOVE CURRY!

BALLS OUT
40–80 SERVINGS

6⅔ pounds Okinawan sweet potatoes, peeled and diced into 1-inch cubes*

6⅔ pounds (baby) carrots

100 stalks cilantro, thoroughly cleaned

5 cups loosely packed Thai basil leaves

8¾ quarts coconut milk

2½ cups sugar

6¼ cups Thai green curry paste

2½ cups freshly squeezed lime juice

5 cups mushroom bouillon

20 tubes silken tofu, cut widthwise into 1-inch-thick discs or 20 (19-ounce) boxes soft tofu, cut into 1-inch cubes

5 quarts cornstarch

Radish sprouts, for garnish

2–4 SERVINGS

⅓ pound Okinawan sweet potatoes, peeled and diced into 1-inch cubes*

⅓ pound (baby) carrots

5 stalks cilantro, thoroughly cleaned

¼ cup loosely packed Thai basil leaves

1¾ cups coconut milk

2 teaspoons sugar

5 tablespoons Thai green curry paste

2 teaspoons freshly squeezed lime juice

¼ cup mushroom bouillon

1 tube silken tofu, cut widthwise into 1-inch-thick discs, or

1 (19-ounce) box soft tofu, cut into 1-inch cubes

1 cup cornstarch

Radish sprouts, for garnish

* Purple potatoes work too but require more time to blanch because of their higher starch content.

1. Bring 2 inches water to a rolling boil in a pot over high heat. In the meantime, fill a large bowl with ice water. When the water boils, cook sweet potatoes for 6–8 minutes. Check to make sure potatoes are cooked through and crunchy, still firm, but not mushy. Remove potatoes (but do not dump the boiling water) and shock in ice water for 2 minutes, or until completely cool to the touch. Remove potatoes, strain, and set aside in a bowl.

2. Next, cook carrots for 4–5 minutes until they are cooked through, crunchy, and firm like the potatoes. Remove carrots and shock in ice water for 2 minutes. Remove carrots, strain, and combine with potatoes.

3. Add cilantro, basil leaves, coconut milk, sugar, and green curry paste to a blender. While blending, add lime juice and mushroom bouillon; blend until you reach a smooth consistency. Set aside.

4. Fill a small pot with 2 inches of oil and bring to 350°F over medium-high heat.

5. Coat tofu with cornstarch (and love) in a bowl, shake off excess starch, then fry tofu for 4–5 minutes, turning over sporadically or until both sides are lightly golden.

6. Remove from oil, shake and discard extra oil into pot, and plate. Garnish with sweet potatoes and carrots.

Heat at least ¾ cup green curry in a pot over medium heat until it simmers. Remove from heat and pour green curry sauce on tofu and vegetables to your heart's desire. Serve with rice.

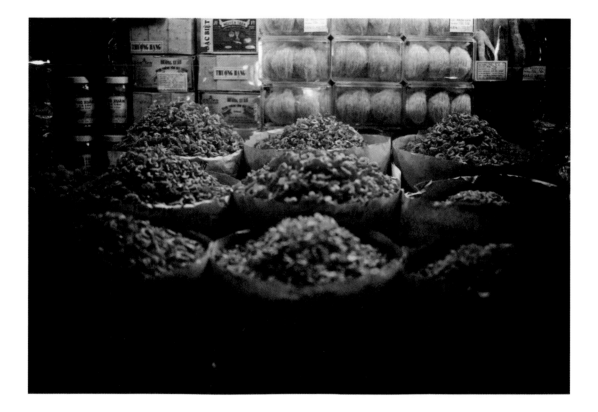

RIBEYE SATAY NOODLES

This dish is not for the average eater. We love this dish, but some (aka many) people don't, even though it is *the* most sent back dish in the history of Starry Kitchen even after I warn them about the funk of (super umami good) dried shrimp. Like I said, not for the average eater, but for those in the know . . . it's not even that funky (it gets way funkier than this in Asia! ha-ha).

2–4 SERVINGS

1⅓ tablespoons minced lemongrass

¾ ounce dried shrimp

¾ heaping teaspoon minced garlic

1 cup Superconcentrated Cantonese Chicken Stock (page 256)

7 tablespoons water

6 tablespoons Coco Rico brand soda

¾ heaping tablespoon creamy peanut butter

6 heaping tablespoons satay (aka sate) sauce

1 teaspoon chicken bouillon (optional)

6 ounces thin pho or rice noodles*

¼ pound ribeye steak, thinly sliced

Kosher salt and pepper

GARNISHES:

2.2 ounces (approximately 2–3 leaves) green leaf lettuce chiffonade

2 tablespoons mint chiffonade

⅓ Persian cucumber, julienned

¼ tomato, thinly sliced

2 tablespoons sesame leaves chiffonade (optional)

Fresh cracked black pepper

¼ lime

* I prefer thinner noodles because you can get all the layers in your mouth, which gives you an amazing texture while you chew. Lots of people like thick rice noodles, and if that's what floats yer boat, who are we to judge?!

BALLS OUT
40–80 SERVINGS

1⅔ cups minced lemongrass

15 ounces dried shrimp

1 cup minced garlic

5 quarts Superconcentrated Cantonese Chicken Stock (page 256)

8¾ cups water

7½ cups Coco Rico brand soda

1 cup creamy peanut butter

7½ cups satay (aka sate) sauce

6⅔ tablespoons chicken bouillon (optional)

7½ pounds pho or rice noodles*

5 pounds ribeye steak, thinly sliced

Kosher salt and pepper

GARNISHES:

2¾ pounds green leaf lettuce chiffonade

2½ cups mint chiffonade

6⅔ Persian cucumbers, julienned

5 tomatoes, thinly sliced

2½ cups sesame leaves chiffonade (optional)

Fresh cracked black pepper

5 whole limes

1. Heat pan/wok with a lil' cooking oil over medium-high heat. With the fervor of an underground chef, sauté and brown the lemongrass, dried shrimp, and garlic, in that order, adding each ingredient after the previous one is finished. Smell the aroma. Take it all in, and transfer your aromatics to a pot. Add chicken stock, water, Coco Rico soda, peanut butter, and satay sauce to that same pot. Mix well, bring to a boil over high heat. Taste, and season accordingly with chicken bouillon as you see fit and remove from heat once it boils.

2. Next, in a separate pot, over high heat boil enough water for your noodles. Once it's at a rolling boil, drop in noodles; start timing the moment they hit the water to track the ideal cook time for the noodles you're using. Parboiled refrigerated pho noodles, our preferred noodle and the kind most pho shops use, take about 2 minutes to boil and get them nice and al dente.

3. Once the noodles are finished, rinse in a colander under cold water to get all the starch off. Shake off excess liquid and arrange in a bowl.

4. Heat pan/wok with some oil over medium-high heat. Lightly season beef with salt and pepper before cooking. When oil starts to lightly smoke, throw in your meat and give both sides a quick sear, but make sure you cook to medium rare. Place on top of noodles.

    Over high heat, boil satay broth. Pour hot satay sauce all over those meatsies to cook them through a little more. Garnish in this order: lettuce, mint, cucumbers, tomatoes, sesame leaves, and some freshly cracked black pepper. Squeeze some lime over all of it, mix it all up, and enjoy . . . the funk!

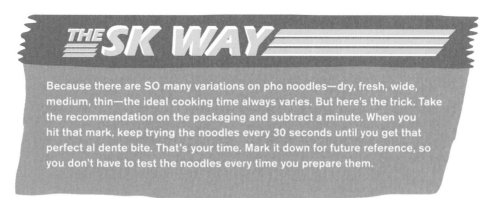

THE SK WAY

Because there are SO many variations on pho noodles—dry, fresh, wide, medium, thin—the ideal cooking time always varies. But here's the trick. Take the recommendation on the packaging and subtract a minute. When you hit that mark, keep trying the noodles every 30 seconds until you get that perfect al dente bite. That's your time. Mark it down for future reference, so you don't have to test the noodles every time you prepare them.

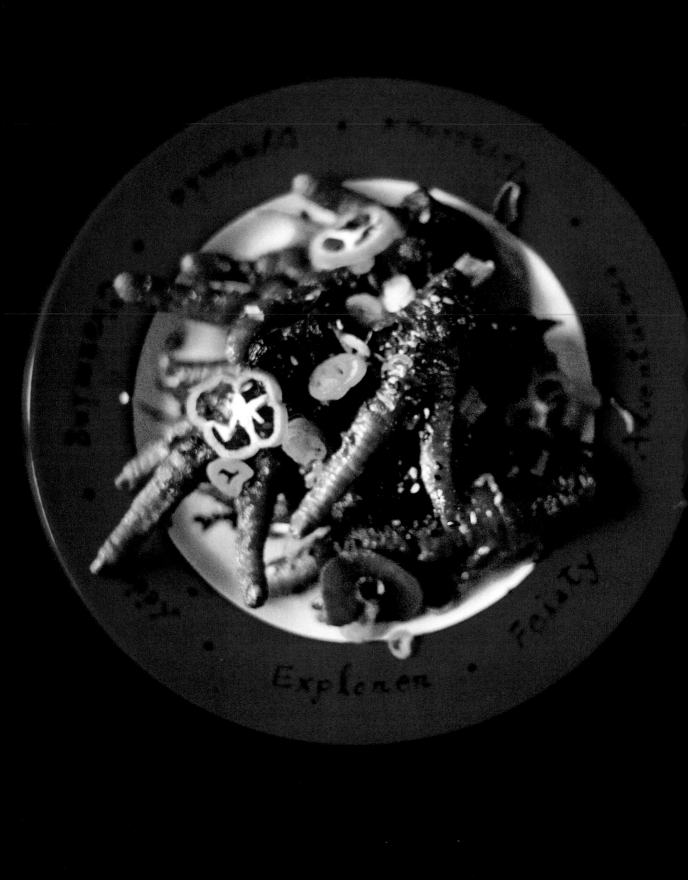

BRAISED SPICY CHICKEN FEET

When the suggestion of eating chicken feet comes up, most (non-Asian, just sayin') people think, "*Eeeeewwwwwwwwwwwww!*" But chicken feet aren't what you might expect. If you're familiar with dim sum, you probably know what to expect. The thing about chicken feet is that they have so few bones. They are almost all cartilage, which takes flavor VERY well, and the collagen gives sauces a naturally thicker consistency. In the end, since there's so little meat . . . ALL you got is deliciously chewy, rich, and saucy FLAVOR.

2–4 SERVINGS

BALLS OUT
40–80 SERVINGS

20 pounds chicken feet

25 star anise pods

60 ounces ginger, sliced

20 scallion stalks, cut into thirds

35 whole dry Thai chili peppers, crushed

5 quarts Superconcentrated Cantonese Chicken Stock (page 256)*

3⅓ cups light soy sauce

10 tablespoons dark soy sauce

1½ cups plus 1 tablespoon oyster sauce

1½ cups plus 1 tablespoon hoisin sauce

5 cinnamon sticks†

1¼ cups sugar

---

1 pound chicken feet

1 star anise pod

3 ounces ginger, sliced

1 scallion stalk, cut into thirds

1¾ whole dry Thai chili peppers, crushed

1 cup Superconcentrated Cantonese Chicken Stock (page 256)*

2⅔ tablespoons light soy sauce

½ tablespoon dark soy sauce

1¼ tablespoons oyster sauce

1¼ tablespoons hoisin sauce

¼ cinnamon stick†

1 tablespoon sugar

Cilantro, for garnish

Scallions, chopped, for garnish

Fresno chilies, small diced or sliced, for garnish

White or black sesame seeds, for garnish

* If you HAVE to, you can use water in this recipe.

† LOVE to use Saigon cinnamon, which (I THINK) is superior cinnamon and brings me great Vietnamese pride.

---

1. Heat 2 inches of oil in a small pot to 350°F.
2. While the oil heats up, clip chicken nails with scissors. Next, rinse chicken feet with cold water in a colander. Drain, then pat dry until the feet are devoid of moisture. If there is any moisture, it will splatter when you fry the feet, which ain't pretty. To make sure the feet are ready to be fried, drip dry them on a plate with towels.
3. In a bowl large enough to hold all the feet, prepare an ice water bath.
4. When the feet are dry and the oil is hot and ready to go, deep-fry chicken feet for about 5–7 minutes until they are a golden brown.

Fry in small enough batches that the oil isn't overcrowded (with feet), because the feet need room to cook.

5. Remove feet from pot, shake off excess oil, drip dry on a plate with a towel for 1 minute, then soak in ice water bath for 1 hour. If the water warms to room temperature, drain and replace with more ice water.

6. Next, drain the bowl completely, then set aside.

7. In a wok/pan, sauté star anise pod, ginger, scallion, and whole chilies with a little bit of cooking oil until the air around you becomes incredibly fragrant. Be careful. If you sauté for too long, the scent can get overwhelmingly powerful.

8. Add chicken feet and stir-fry for 1 minute, then combine with stock, light soy sauce, dark soy sauce, oyster sauce, hoisin sauce, cinnamon stick, and sugar.

9. Bring to a boil over high heat. Once it boils, lower heat and let simmer for 45 minutes, or until chicken feet are tender.

10. Once the feet are tender, remove feet, set aside on a plate or bowl, and return the same pot to a boil over medium-high heat for 5–10 minutes and reduce sauce to a thicker consistency.

Remove from heat and discard the cinnamon stick. Chicken feet are far more tasty if cooled to room temperature, placed back into the thickened sauce pot, covered, and refrigerated overnight so all the flavor seeps deep into them. When you're ready to serve, reheat in sauce over medium-high heat for 7–10 minutes, then plate with plenty of sauce drizzled on top (or extra sauce in a bowl) and garnish with cilantro, scallions, Fresno chilies, and sesame seeds. Chew away!

SHRIMP AND PORK CHILI OIL WONTONS WITH SZECHUAN SHREDDED POTATOES

Categorically speaking (on Yelp), we're considered an "Asian fusion" restaurant. I used to be real uppity and kind of snooty about that—"Oh NO, we're not fancy FU-SION!" Although I've since come to terms with that, I still prefer saying we're a "pan-Asian" or an "Asian-Asian" restaurant. Yeah, I know it's quirky and doesn't make sense—until you come across a dish like THIS, which is the marriage of two popular Szechuan (Sichuan) dishes that just make sense to fuse = Asian-Asian fusion.

2–4 SERVINGS

SZECHUAN CHILI OIL:

10 tablespoons chili oil

6½ tablespoons light soy sauce

2½ tablespoons sugar

10 tablespoons Superconcentrated Cantonese Chicken Stock (page 256)

5 teaspoons minced garlic

WONTONS:

2 russet potatoes, peeled and thinly julienned

2 ounces fresh ginger

6½ ounces shrimp, head-off, peeled, and deveined (see The SK Way, p. 144)

1 pound ground pork

2 teaspoons sesame oil

2 teaspoons Chinese cooking wine

6 strands green or yellow chives

1 tablespoon chicken bouillon

3 pinches ground black pepper

3 pinches ground white pepper

1 teaspoon kosher salt

1 large egg

1 pack wonton wrappers*

4 dried whole Thai chili peppers

¼ red bell pepper, julienned

3 tablespoons rice vinegar

2 pinches kosher salt

2 pinches sugar

Scallion, finely chopped, for garnish

* We like our wrappers thin and chewy, with a visible amount of powdery starch in the pack, which usually means the wrappers are made fresh and the wrappers aren't stuck together.

BALLS OUT
40–80 SERVINGS

SZECHUAN CHILI OIL:

7 cups tablespoons chili oil

4½ cups light soy sauce

1½ cups sugar

7 cups Superconcentrated Cantonese Chicken Stock (page 256)

1 cup garlic, minced

WONTONS:

20 russet potatoes, peeled and thinly julienned

1¼ pounds fresh ginger

4 pounds shrimp

10 pounds ground pork

¼ cup sesame oil

¼ cup Chinese cooking wine

12 ounces green or yellow chives

10 tablespoons chicken bouillon

1¾ teaspoons ground black pepper

1¾ teaspoons ground white pepper

3½ tablespoons kosher salt

10 large eggs

10 packs wonton wrappers*

40 dried whole Thai chili peppers

2¼ red bell pepper, julienned

1¾ cups rice vinegar

1¼ teaspoons kosher salt

1¼ teaspoons sugar

1. **MAKE YOUR SZECHUAN CHILI OIL FIRST:** Mix all chili oil ingredients in a pot and heat until sugar dissolves. Remove from heat and cool to room temperature before using or refrigerating (covered).
2. Soak potatoes in a salted ice water bath to remove starch (this is the same thing we do for our airy and crunchy french fries).
3. Crush ginger with the flat side of a cleaver or a dull end of any object. Soak in a bowl of cold water for 3–4 minutes.
4. Hand-mince shrimp with a knife until the texture is slightly chunky. Transfer to a larger mixing bowl to combine all the wonton wrapping ingredients.
5. Check on potatoes. If water is too cloudy, drain and refill bowl with more ice water.
6. Next, in the bowl with the shrimp, add ground pork, sesame oil, cooking wine, chives, chicken bouillon, black pepper, white pepper, and salt. Mix thoroughly with your hands in one direction until the mix is fully incorporated.
7. Remove ginger from water and dispose of the ginger; then slowly incorporate ginger-infused water into the pork-shrimp mix. Make sure meat fully absorbs the water. Cover and refrigerate for 30 minutes.
8. Drain water from the potato bowl; to get those potatoes extra crunchy, wash and shake off remaining starch under a constant stream of cold water until the water is completely clear. To prevent oxidization, leave potatoes submerged in water; set aside until ready to cook.
9. When ready to wrap your wontons, beat egg for your egg wash in a separate bowl. Set aside.
10. Remove pork-shrimp mixture from refrigerator. Wrap your wontons on a clean and flat work surface (either a countertop or a large cutting board) that has been dusted with all-purpose flour. This will prevent any sticking or drying out while wrapping. Sprinkle on more flour as needed.
11. Open wonton wrapper packaging and fully cover wrappers with a damp towel; keep them covered at all times to prevent drying out and/or unraveling. Unused wrappers can be refrigerated for two or three days.
12. Next, lay down a single wonton wrapper and position it like a diamond. In the center of the diamond, place about a teaspoon of pork-shrimp mixture, roughly the size of a quarter.

13. Spread a thin layer of egg wash across the top corner of the wrapper. Bring together the bottom and top corners of the wrapper, pinch them together, then pinch along and seal both diagonal edges down to the side corners, forming a wonton triangle. Then fold in side corners one after the other so they overlap. Lightly pinch the folded side corners together so that they stick to one another. Place wrapped wontons on a tray. Repeat for the rest of the wontons.

14. Next, bring 2 inches of water to a boil over high heat.

15. While waiting for the water to boil, remove potatoes from water, pat dry, and set aside.

16. Next, dry-roast dried chili peppers in a pan/wok over high heat for 1 minute, then set aside in a bowl. Sauté bell peppers with a little cooking oil for 2 minutes, or until they're cooked through but still crunchy. Set aside in a different bowl.

17. Stir-fry potatoes with cooking oil for 2–3 minutes. Then add rice vinegar, salt, and sugar. Continue stir-frying until the potatoes are slightly translucent, but still crunchy. Hand-break roasted chilies into the pan, quickly toss in, remove pan from heat, plate, and top with the sautéed bell peppers and scallions.

18. Once water starts boiling, add wontons to pot and cook for 5–8 minutes. Give your wontons enough space to swim freely. Don't pack them too tightly in the pot of water. To make sure the filling is cooked through, bite into one or check the internal temperature, which should be 145°F or higher.

    Remove wontons from water with a slotted spoon, plate on top of stir-fried potatoes, and liberally ladle as much Szechuan Chili Oil on top of the wontons and enough for the potatoes to swim in a shallow pool of chili flavor. Enjoy while trying to get every little bit in every bite . . . the potato, bell pepper, and wonton. It's an amazing marriage of flavor and textures. Enjoy feasting on our fusion!

We knew nothing about running a restaurant.

—FAILURES

SESAME OIL SPARERIBS

Slow-roasted ribs from our marijuana dinners . . . *sans* marijuana, but still delicious. Need I write more?

BALLS OUT
40–80 SERVINGS

RIBS:

¾ cup plus
1⅓ tablespoons tapioca
starch

120 spareribs,
individually cut

1¼ cups oyster sauce

½ cup plus 2 tablespoons
light soy sauce

6⅔ tablespoons
sesame oil

10 tablespoons freshly
grated ginger juice*

1⅔ tablespoons black
pepper

WRAPPING:

60 pieces angelica root,
halved

2½ cups goji berries (aka
wolfberries)

120 small sprigs cilantro

2–4 SERVINGS

RIBS:

2 teaspoons tapioca
starch

6 spareribs,
individually cut

1 tablespoon oyster
sauce

½ tablespoon light soy
sauce

1 teaspoon sesame oil

½ tablespoon freshly
grated ginger juice*

¼ teaspoon black
pepper

WRAPPING:

3 pieces angelica root,
halved

2 tablespoons goji
berries (aka wolfberries)

6 small sprigs cilantro

* Just grate ginger, and
you'll get juice—it's
that simple . . . except
it takes a TEENY bit of
work

---

1. In a bowl, sprinkle and dry-rub tapioca starch onto ribs.
2. In a separate bowl, mix oyster sauce, light soy sauce, sesame oil, ginger juice, and black pepper. Immerse ribs in the mixed sauce and rub sauce onto every inch of every part of every rib.
3. Cover and refrigerate for at least 1 hour, but we highly recommend marinating overnight for the most amazing flavor and texture.
4. When ready, preheat oven to 350°F. Remove ribs from fridge, remove from bowl, and lay out on a sheet of aluminum foil with enough foil to fully envelop the ribs. Fold up edges into a large pouch, but do not close. Add angelica root, goji berries, cilantro, and then wrap up ribs in foil.
5. Place wrapped ribs onto the middle rack of oven. Cook for 1½ hours, check, and roast until desired tenderness is achieved. We recommend a balance between moist and almost-falling-off-the-bone-but-not-quite because ribs are really fun to eat with your hands.
6. Once fully roasted, remove from oven and transfer to a bowl/plate with foil wrapping intact.

    When ready to serve, open foil and eat with your favorite starch.

MARIJUANA— A MEAL FOR ONE AND ALL

I WAS A SOMEWHAT NARC-ISH WEIRD KID WHO WANTED TO FEEL LIKE THE NORMAL "OTHER KIDS." EVEN THROUGH HIGH SCHOOL, I WAS PRETTY STRAITLACED: I PREACHED ABSTINENCE BEFORE MARRIAGE (WHAT A WASTED OPPORTUNITY); I DIDN'T DO DRUGS OR DRINK; I WENT BACK TO MY CATHOLIC CHURCH TO GET CONFIRMED; I DIDN'T MASTURBATE, YA KNOW. I WANTED TO BE THE KIND OF PERSON SOCIETY DEEMED "GOOD," AND I SOMEHOW CAME TO THIS CONCLUSION AS A TEENAGER ON MY OWN, WITH A LOT OF HELP FROM ALL THE "DON'T DO DRUGS" BRAIN-WASHING, GROWING UP IN THE BUCKLE OF THE BIBLE BELT, SELF-MOTIVATION (AND SELF-DENIAL—SO, SO, SO MUCH SELF-DENIAL), AND, OF COURSE, PRETTY CRIPPLING ISSUES CONCERNING MY CULTURAL IDENTITY AND IMAGE. IT'S EASY TO BE GOOD, I SUPPOSE, WHEN YOU BELIEVE YOU'RE NOT A NORMAL KID OR PART OF THE COOL GROUP. I WAS A BOY SCOUT, LITERALLY AND FIGURATIVELY. (OKAY, I'M LYING. I DROPPED OUT OF CUB SCOUTS, BUT STILL, I WAS A BOY SCOUT IN THE AMERICAN CULTURAL SENSE.)

Which is the natural progression into . . . hosting marijuana dinners as an adult!

Now I'll backtrack by confirming how weird I am as an adult. A lot of times, we as adults overcompensate for things we feel we lost out on in our childhoods or things we felt inadequate about. (That's at least what I've gathered from listening to decades of Dr. Drew and taking a prelim psyche class—I'm almost an expert, ya know.) So now we've laid the groundwork for that—SET!

Next point: I like weed (aka marijuana, if that vernacular is lost on anyone who is in the weird-Nguyen-Tran-in-high-school phase), but I'm not a fiend for it. I don't need it. I smoke it once or twice a year, and only because someone else has it and I didn't have to pay for it (SCORE) and/or didn't have to pick through

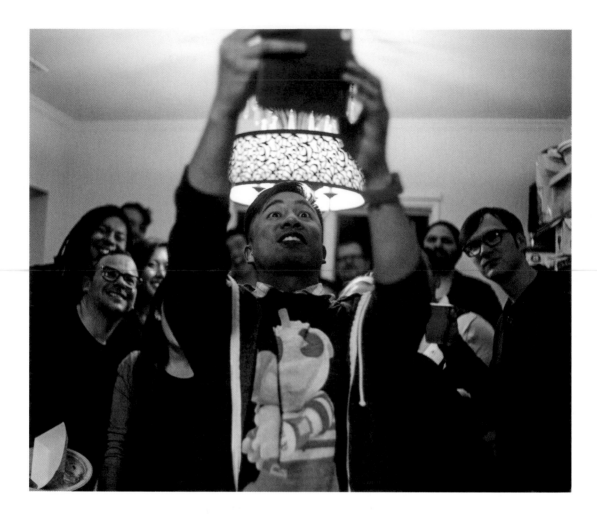

the bud and roll it myself (DOUBLE SCORE, because I really don't know how to do that . . . see, I'm NOT a pothead!). I don't crave it. But I sure don't mind it.

During Starry Kitchen's lunch brick-and-mortar days, we occasionally hosted these not-so-fancy-but-kinda-fancy French food pop-ups with Laurent Quenioux (aka LQ), a locally acclaimed chef and an absolute beast in the kitchen. LQ had just closed down his own restaurant, Bistro LQ, and I figured, what would be crazier and more unexpected than French chef LQ bringing his food to our not-so-fancy food court space and my Starry Kitchen craziness! It worked, and word spread fast. We got lots of press about our collaboration (which is honestly the wrong word because it was almost *all* LQ, but once in a blue moon I would chime in with a pretty good idea), including the time we hosted a nineteen-course white truffle menu. Oh man, I still remember shelling out thousands of dollars for those white truffles. So deep in aroma. So deep in flavor. So . . . deep in debt because those little chunks of an earthy-rich mushroom cost so much. I mean, it's kinda worth it, but still damn expensive, y'all. Three thousand dollars for one pound—that's a lot to me, and if I ever become more rich with actual money than culture, I'm still going to think that's expensive as fuck!

Once we had accomplished the nineteen courses of A-grade white truffles dinner, I thought we could take on the world. So I goaded LQ that we should do something crazier. LQ half-jokingly suggested a marijuana dinner.

Now, I don't know whether I'm like other people (I MIGHT not be), but sometimes I get a feeling that the stars are perfectly aligned; Mercury isn't in retrograde; the Earth is spinning at exactly the correct angle on its axis; the air is at the right density; and somewhere in the city, Shia Labeouf is staging more life-changing, frighteningly serious, deeply hilarious, and never anything short of purely amazing exhibitionist art—and THAT is what I felt like at the sheer mention of doing a marijuana dinner. The idea hit a bulls-eye deep in my soul. I KNEW it had to happen, though LQ was a little scared.

It required deep planning, and by "planning" I do NOT mean sitting around and smoking a shitload of weed until someone had enough of the munchies to start cooking. NO, actual *adult* planning. Adulting ain't easy for me, but I accept it as a cost of releasing my inner man-child to play. LQ was adamant about making this much classier than people might expect, as he did not want to be labeled a marijuana chef. LQ and Thi agreed on making

the event a Chinese herb and marijuana dinner. Or as I like to call it, the "Take-things-that-normally-taste-like-shit-and-make-them-taste-good dinner!"

To prepare for the dinner, Thi did a tremendous amount of research about Traditional Chinese Medicine, flavor profile, anatomical responses, and the marriage with marijuana, which a long time ago was considered to be part of the Chinese medicine family until some knucklehead made it illegal, ruining the fun for everyone.

We brainstormed fun ways how *not* to get busted. LQ definitely didn't want to get busted or have someone try to deport him—even though he's a U.S. citizen. And, although she was already deeply kinda-sorta "part" of the illegal+underground Starry Kitchen ways, Thi meant it when she told me, "If you get arrested, I'm breaking up with your ass."

If I were personally scared of getting caught for doing anything that isn't the norm, we would never have started Starry Kitchen in the first place. So everyone, EVERYONE, had to sign a contract waiver stating that they deferred all responsibility to me (only MOI!), which gave them plausible deniability. Basically, "This Is All Nguyen Tran's Fault" is probably the best way to summarize the waiver. Which made me the "Kingpin," the Tony Montana of the marijuana dinner—and yes, like Tony Montana, I'm far too in love with myself, and I completely relished that fact, and everyone around me was more calm believing that only I would go to jail if we got caught.

In all of this, we agreed that getting people high was NOT the point. Anyone could get high for much cheaper on their own, which meant that the level of marijuana/THC in the food had to be pretty low and balanced with flavors that would still bring out the essence of the marijuana. Naturally, I volunteered for the important task of taste-testing, paying attention to how long it took to get high (taking hits for the team is what I do—am I not a kind and generous megalomaniac?). Those were awkward calls because I would be really happy; my reaction time was notably very slow and then I'd be like, "I feel great, but we still gotta lower the THC in this—okay, I'm gonna get some jalapeño cheddar Cheetos and check ya later!"

We also agreed that the location had to be secret. So secret that we didn't even share with the staff the address of where we were cooking until the day of the dinners in order to protect them and keep the information from getting out.

The secret goal of the first marijuana dinner was simple: to have the perfect dinner party. I didn't want only potheads; I didn't want only rich people. I wanted people from all walks of life, a great balance of gender, ideology, humor, and, most important, people who were openly creative.

To make sure I invited the right people, I made everyone, and I mean EVERYONE, take a personality test. Even nationally known and respected food critic Jonathan Gold had to take the test. There were ridiculous questions like "If you were a potato chip, what kind would you be?"—questions designed to "weed out" the douchebags. From the answers to those fun

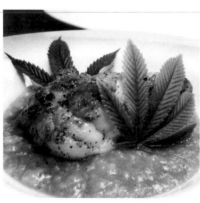

questions, I got a feel for how a person would act. Would that person be interesting? Would she have something to contribute? Would he be fun to hang out with?

I got hundreds of applications and I pored over every single one of them to identify the thirty most unique candidates for this special occasion. People were elated, paid for their meal, and waited for the update containing the secret details.

In homage to *The Simpsons,* we called the event the "Grammar Rodeo" after the hilarious episode "Bart on the Road," about the road trip of a lifetime. I wrote a detailed email about how (seriously) excited we were about everyone's involvement in that year's Grammar Rodeo, what to expect, and that we'd be offering a free and purely optional special dinner, in Starry Kitchen's proud illegal+underground standard operating procedure, if anyone wanted to hang around.

I also included in the email the strictest of rules: The minute the last course was done, everyone had to get the FUCK out! We knew that no matter what, with enough THC in our guests' systems, they would get high. It was never a question of if, but when—and then what? We most definitely didn't want to be around when our guests got high because we'd never be able to get them out of the secret location.

We picked everyone up at a random grocery store. I arrived in a nondescript van, designed to look like any other film or TV production transport van in LA, with a "Grammar Rodeo" sign taped inside the windshield. To disorient people so they couldn't figure out where we were, I drove the longest way possible and did what I do best—TALKED nonstop to distract everyone.

I also forbade anyone from posting on social media during the dinner, lest we got caught. I wasn't about to let someone inadvertently narc on us and ruin the night for everyone. It was also a good reminder that we were all IN CA-HOOTS, which made the event even more fun.

The dinner was a huge success. Two special guests—Jonathan Gold, the Pulitzer Prize–winning food "poet" reviewer, and Elise McDonough, of *High Times* magazine—were announced at the dinner as a surprise. When crazy serious foodies saw and recognized Jonathan Gold, they went nuts. But once I introduced Elise to a room of partial potheads, Jonathan played second fiddle to the woman who had brought joy to so many people in the room through an herb that brought them immensely more joy and relaxation than had ever been known to the world. Nostalgia always wins out in a battle of celebrity!

The night went by quickly. Nine courses, all plated in a beautiful single-story home in Encino (another part of the puzzle—in LA,

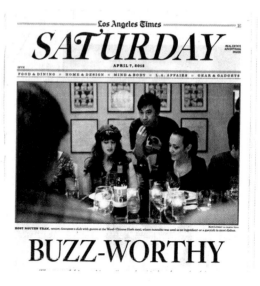

NOTHING cool ever happens in the Valley, so that felt like the most natural place to have this dinner). Music, food, conversation, people reminiscing about when and how they first got high, and some people watching a runner who admitted that he had never gotten high before—to monitor his reactions.

Mystery. Wonderment. A special event that only the people in that room got to experience. Right after dessert, we directed everyone to the front door, handed them a special chocolate in a jar of marijuana mist, and took people back to the grocery store in waves to end the night.

The secret goal of the marijuana dinner was simple: to have the perfect dinner party.

OSMANTHUS PANNA COTTA W/ RED WINE POACHED PEARS

Thi doesn't like to publicly admit this, but the Osmanthus Panna Cotta is actually one of her favorite desserts, maybe because it was originally conceived for our marijuana dinners. There's no marijuana in this recipe, but if you want to add it, I'm not going to stop you. Start with a cannabis-infused oil or fat and mix it with tapioca maltodextrin, which, despite its delicate, gastronomical-sounding name, will powderize your fat. Garnish with that "soil powder" and—voilà!—a marijuana-infused dessert.

BALLS OUT
40–80 SERVINGS

RED WINE POACHED PEARS:

15 Green Anjou pears, peeled and each cut into 6 pieces

5 (750ml) bottles red wine

5 cups sugar

5 cinnamon sticks

5 star anise pods

1⅔ tablespoons vanilla extract

OSMANTHUS PANNA COTTA:

9 tablespoons gelatin powder, or 27 bronze gelatin sheets/leaves

9 cups heavy whipping cream

9 cups whole milk

6 ¾ tablespoons osmanthus flower*

2¼ cups sugar

2–4 SERVINGS

RED WINE POACHED PEARS:

3 Green Anjou pears, peeled and each cut into 6 pieces

1 (750ml) bottle red wine

1 cup sugar

1 cinnamon stick

1 star anise pod

1 teaspoon vanilla extract

OSMANTHUS PANNA COTTA:

1 tablespoon gelatin powder, or 3 bronze gelatin sheets/leaves

⅓ cup plus ⅔ cup heavy whipping cream

1 cup whole milk

2¼ teaspoons osmanthus flower*

¼ cup sugar

Red Wine Poached Pears, for garnish

* This is readily available in traditional Chinese medicine (TCM) shops or Asian grocery stores with a TCM section.

1. **FOR THE RED WINE POACHED PEARS:** Take note of how ripe the pears are before starting. The riper the pear, the shorter the cooking time.

2. Combine wine, sugar, cinnamon, star anise, and vanilla extract in a saucepan or pot. Boil over high heat and mix until sugar dissolves. Lower to medium heat, add pears, cover, and poach for 3–4 minutes, making sure pears stay submerged. Cooking time will vary depending on the ripeness of the pears.

3. To test for doneness, pierce a piece of pear (I absolutely adore alliteration!). It should be tender all the way through. If not, cook a little bit longer and test again.

4. Remove pears from pot; let them cool in a bowl or on a plate.

5. Continue boiling the wine mixture to reduce by half the original volume, or until it takes on a more syrupy consistency. Remove from

heat and let cool to room temperature. Transfer pears back to wine reduction, cover and store in refrigerator until ready to serve.

6. **FOR THE PANNA COTTA:** If using gelatin sheets, add to a bowl of ice-cold water and submerge. Soak (aka let them bloom) for 5–7 minutes, or until they soften. To prevent sheets from breaking down, drain water immediately after the 5–7 minutes and gently wring out remaining water from the sheets, just like you were wringing out a towel.

7. If using powdered gelatin, place gelatin in a bowl and add ⅓ cup heavy cream (or more, to completely dissolve, if needed). Let it sit. Let it bloom.

8. If using a fun mold to shape and pop out your panna cotta, brush a light layer of cooking oil on the bottom and sides.

9. Combine remaining heavy cream, milk, and osmanthus flower in a pot and bring to a simmer over medium heat. Remove from heat and cover for 10 minutes to infuse the osmanthus.

10. After the osmanthus has infused, strain and dispose of the flowers. Add sugar to pot over medium-low heat and stir until sugar dissolves and liquid steams, but not boils. If you have a thermometer, DO NOT go over 145°F.

11. Next, add gelatin (sheets or powdered in heavy cream), then whisk until gelatin dissolves. This will take a few minutes.

12. Remove from heat and mix gently with a spatula.

13. Ladle into ramekins, small bowls, or your preferred fancy or not-so-fancy container, or into your pre-oil-brushed mold.

14. Refrigerate, carefully. Gelatin is fairly docile and irritably unstable. As it cools, however, panna cotta should solidify within an hour.

15. Garnish with poached pears on top, and drizzle the red wine sauce all over and any other fancy way you want to have fun with the canvas that is your plate. (*swoosh*)

SEPARATION TIP: If your chilled panna cotta separates into layers of milk and cream, it's because the mixture wasn't adequately whisked or sometimes because it was too warm when you introduced the gelatin. To avoid this, let the mixture come to room temperature, then whisk again and pour back into the cups or molds.

PANDAN BAVARIAN CREAM

Our obsession with pandan is almost unparalleled. We love everything about it—the *Pandanus am-aryllifolius* plant it comes from, the green hue it gives to dishes, and the sense of whimsy it inspires in people clearly eating with their eyes. We are but simple subjects of this alluring substitute for vanilla in Southeast Asia. Inspired by a former cook of ours, we decided to make it so we could allit-eratively say we served Pandan Profiteroles ... oh, and also because they're delish! #pandan4ever

BALLS OUT
40–80 SERVINGS

1¼ cups plus 3¾ cups cold water

1¼ cups powdered gelatin

5 quarts heavy whipping cream

40 large egg yolks

5 quarts milk

5 cups sugar

1¼ teaspoons kosher salt

3⅓ tablespoons pure vanilla extract

2½ teaspoons pandan extract

2–4 SERVINGS

2 tablespoons plus 6 tablespoons cold water

2 tablespoons powdered gelatin

2 cups heavy whipping cream

4 large egg yolks

2 cups milk

½ cup sugar

1 pinch kosher salt

1 teaspoon pure vanilla extract

¼ teaspoon pandan extract

1. Add 2 tablespoons cold water to a bowl large enough to hold all the water in this recipe; sprinkle in gelatin and whisk until gelatin dis-solves. Let it sit for 5 minutes, or until mixture gels.
2. Next, bring the remainder of the water to a simmer in a pot over medium-high heat. Once it simmers, remove from heat and pour this water into the gelatin mix bowl. Whisk until fully incorporated. Set aside.
3. Pour heavy cream into another bowl and whisk until stiff peaks of whipped cream start to form. Cover and refrigerate.
4. Beat egg yolks in a separate bowl, large enough to hold the eggs and milk. Set aside.
5. Next, heat milk, sugar, and salt in a new pot/pan on medium heat, whisking occasionally, until milk starts to steam. Then slowly com-bine that milk mix in the bowl of beaten egg yolks and whisk till completely mixed in. Pour back into the pot and bring to a simmer over low heat for 2 minutes, stirring frequently.
6. Remove from heat. Now stir in the dissolved gelatin, vanilla extract, and pandan extract to start forming the Bavarian cream.
7. Strain Bavarian cream mixture twice through a chinois or fine mesh

sieve and pour into a bowl. Next, fill one-third of a large bowl with ice water. (This bowl needs to be large enough to hold the water and the bowl full of the Bavarian cream without spilling over.) Gently nestle the Bavarian cream bowl in the ice water bath, making sure the ice water doesn't overflow into the cream. With a hand mixer or by hand, beat the cream until it cools and starts to thicken. Then gently fold the refrigerated whipped cream into the Bavarian cream by adding large glops of whipped cream and folding them in, one at a time.

Store, cover, and refrigerate for 3 hours, pipe it into the profiteroles, your favorite pastries, or enjoy however you want.

Starry Kitchen is the
Ultimate Move by My Wife
to Shut Me the Fuck Up!

—KITCHEN NINJA

PROFITEROLES

These Profiteroles are a perfect example of how obsessive we can be. But instead of detailing the months we spent on making, remaking, and reliving the not-always-pleasant neurotic memories of this one recipe (and honestly for a lot of recipes), let's just get y'all closer to making this and piping in that Pandan Bavarian Cream you patiently made yourself!

BALLS OUT
40–80 SERVINGS

7½ cups water

3¾ cups unsalted butter, cut into ½-inch slices

5 tablespoons sugar

1¼ teaspoons kosher salt

7½ cups flour

30 plus 10 large eggs

2–4 SERVINGS

¾ cup water	1½ teaspoons sugar	3 plus 1 large eggs
6 tablespoons unsalted butter, cut into ½-inch slices	2 pinches kosher salt	
	¾ cup flour	

1. Preheat oven to 400°F.
2. Line a baking sheet with parchment paper or a silicone baking mat (aka Silpat mat—they're GREAT), or lightly line a pan with brushed-on melted butter. Sprinkle flour across it. Set aside.
3. Next, combine water, butter, sugar, and salt in a pot/pan. Bring to a boil over medium-high heat and stir until butter completely melts. Lower to medium heat and add flour and stir until dough pulls away from sides of pan and forms a ball. Remove from heat and let it cool for 10 minutes.
4. Transfer dough into a stand mixer, if you have one, or a mixing bowl, if you don't. Fold three eggs into the dough, one at a time. Mix with paddle attachment or by hand with a rubber spatula.
5. Transfer the dough into piping bag, then pipe as many 1½-inch-long strands of dough onto your lined baking sheet as you can. Leave about 2 inches between each strand.
6. Beat the remaining egg in a separate bowl, then brush egg wash over all the dough strands. This step ensures a nice crunchy top for the profiterole. Transfer the baking sheet to the middle rack of the oven and bake for 20 minutes. Reduce temperature to 350°F and bake for an additional 10 minutes, or until the profiteroles are golden brown.

Next, use a skewer or similar tool to pierce a hole in one end of each pastry to allow steam to escape and, later, to pipe in the cream. Continue to bake for 5 minutes.

Remove profiteroles from oven and let cool on a rack. Pipe in your Pandan Bavarian Cream or whatever other deliciousness your heart and mouth desire. Enjoy!

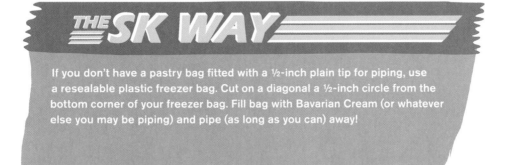

THE SK WAY

If you don't have a pastry bag fitted with a ½-inch plain tip for piping, use a resealable plastic freezer bag. Cut on a diagonal a ½-inch circle from the bottom corner of your freezer bag. Fill bag with Bavarian Cream (or whatever else you may be piping) and pipe (as long as you can) away!

SALTED DUCK EGG CEREAL PRAWNS

This is the beautiful marriage of two seemingly different but incredibly delicious Singaporean dishes—cereal prawns and butter prawns. Fresh curry leaves and HUGE shell-on prawns make for a TRUE finger lickin'ly memorable get-down-and-dirty experience. Same-culture fusion at its finest. It should have happened sooner, and it's happening for you now.

BALLS OUT
40–80 SERVINGS

90 large (7½ pounds, U12) whole shell-on prawns

Kosher salt and black pepper

2¾ cups cornstarch

45 cloves garlic, coarsely chopped

30 Thai chilies, sliced into rings

15 Fresno chilies, sliced into rings

45 sprigs fresh curry leaves

2 cups unsalted butter

30 salted duck egg yolks*

2¾ quarts and 1 quart instant/dry Singaporean breakfast cereal flakes

5 tablespoons chicken bouillon

2¾ teaspoons sugar

2–4 SERVINGS

6 large (½ pound, U12) whole shell-on prawns

Kosher salt and black pepper

3 tablespoons cornstarch

3 cloves garlic, coarsely chopped

2 Thai chilies, sliced into rings

1 Fresno chili, sliced into rings

3 sprigs fresh curry leaves

2 tablespoons unsalted butter

2 salted duck egg yolks*

¾ cup and ¼ cup instant/dry Singaporean breakfast cereal flakes (Nestum or similar)

1 teaspoon chicken bouillon

2 pinches sugar

Cilantro, roughly chopped, for garnish

* These are typically sold in small cartons as whole eggs. We try to buy eggs sourced from Taiwan.

1. Thaw out prawns. Once thawed, use a pair of scissors to remove legs, then split the shell by cutting along the back from the tail to just short of the head. Next, slit the back of the prawn's body with a knife. Look out for a black vein. If it's there, remove it and devein the prawn. Leave the head and shell intact.
2. Rinse and pat the prawns dry. Season with salt and pepper. Lightly coat prawns in bowl with cornstarch. Remove, shake off excess, set aside on a plate or in another bowl.
3. Heat 2 inches of cooking oil in a pot to 350°F over high heat. Once the oil is hot enough, completely submerge the prawns and deep-fry for 3–4 minutes, or until fully cooked and crispy. Remove and shake off excess oil. Set aside.
4. In a saucepan under medium-high heat, sauté garlic, Thai and Fresno chilies, and curry leaves in butter until evenly browned. The air

should turn fragrant, and your hangover from the night before should be completely gone. YAY! Add salted egg yolks. Crush them, stir, then reduce to medium heat.

5. Add ¾ cup cereal. Stir until the flakes look and smell roasted. Add the rest of the cereal and combine until ingredients are dried up. Add chicken bouillon and sugar. Mix, taste, and adjust seasoning to your liking.

6. Toss in prawns. Continue to stir-fry until prawns are well-coated.

Remove from heat. Plate and garnish with cilantro. To eat, dig in with your fingers because there's no time to be dainty here. Go at it (shells, head-on and all)—like no one is watching!

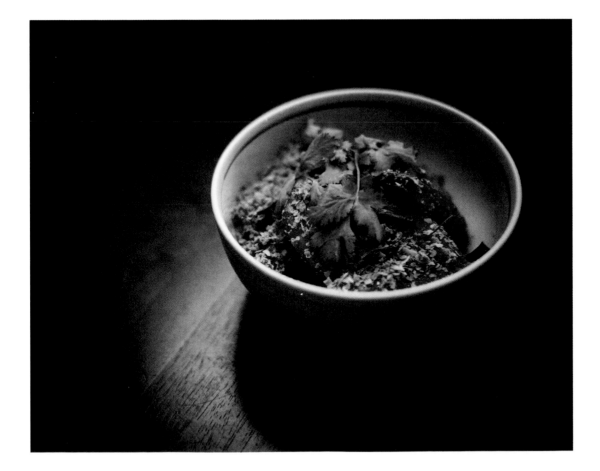

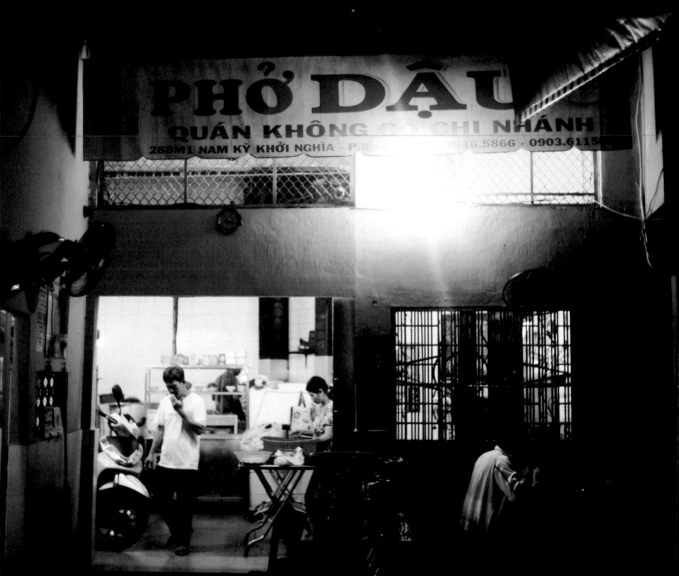

GROWING UP ASIAN

CONTRARY TO MY CURRENT REPUTATION, I WAS ONCE THE ULTRA-QUIET AND INORDINATELY SHY SPAWN OF MY YOUNG AND LOVING PARENTS. THEY WERE ONLY TEENAGERS WHEN THEY FLED VIETNAM AT THE END OF THE WAR AND LANDED IN NOT-YET-GENTRIFIED FAIRFAX, VIRGINIA. I WAS SIX MONTHS OLD WHEN THE GOOD OL' 'RENTS MOVED THE FAM TO HOT, HOT DALLAS, TEXAS, WHERE I SPENT ALL OF MY FORMATIVE YEARS.

Being a kid is hard enough. But being a Vietnamese kid in a predominantly white neighborhood—in 1980s Texas, no less—was two doors down from impossible. Most kids (THIS kid included) don't want to stand out. They want to be part of the club. Part of the pack. Not a weirdo. This ain't happening when you're a diaspora kid, a kid of hyphenated descent: a Chinese-American kid, an Armenian-American kid, or in my case, a Vietnamese-American kid. You're always going to stand out (at least where I grew up). It's just the way it is.

On top of not being "normal," we hyphenated kids suffer the double misfortune of having to straddle two cultures: one that doesn't want anything to do with us, and another faraway culture that we don't feel connected to in any significant way. Growing up in Dallas, I didn't want to be seen as Vietnamese. I didn't want to be considered the "other" kid. I wanted to be seen as an American, as American as J. R. Ewing, Magnum P. I., and Alex P. Keaton—or any other white male with initials attached to his American-sounding name. American. Period. No hyphens. I wanted to be white, desperately so, and no amount of white-washing could satisfy my desire to fit in.

But my classmates made sure that that was never going to happen. They bullied me, taunted me, and tagged me, in the geographic and cultural ignorance of the region, as a "Chinese kid." They pronounced my name wrong. They made fun of the food my parents served at home and packed in my metal Pac-Man lunchbox (until I convinced my parents not to send any more weird food with me). Because I wanted to fit in, I wanted to each Lunchables like everyone else, I made fun of the food my parents grew up on, too, telling my classmates every chance I got, "Yeah, I don't eat THAT food. It's gross!" For most of the first eighteen years of my life, I resisted, and then almost rejected entirely, Vietnamese food, deciding it was in my best interest to devour hamburgers and hotdogs and chips and queso like a madman—an *American* madman.

One time, the local equivalent of *Parade* magazine interviewed my mom about her life as a refugee, growing up in Vietnam and then assimilating into American culture. My mom mentioned to the reporter that her cute and adorable son was as American as could be. "He only eats hamburgers and hotdogs," she said. Oh man!—outed by my mom, thrown under the diaspora bus rolling down the bumpy road to assimilation. Sure, I wanted to be American, but I also wanted the praise and love of my parents, and I knew even then that they wanted me to respect my Vietnamese roots, to practice the customs and celebrate the culture and cuisine of their homeland. But I didn't know how to connect with that part of myself. I didn't understand it. Why did I have to cross my arms every time I entered the homes of elders and greet them? Why did I have to do the same thing when I said goodbye? I said "Hi," didn't I?! Why did I have to take my shoes off? Why did I have to acknowledge all elders individually when I barely knew who they were? Why did we have to take something to everyone's home when they invited us over? Why did I have to bother with ANY OF THIS?!

Honestly, my mother's words hurt me deeper than I realized. I was *almost* ashamed, because I was supposed to be this Vietnamese kid, and I didn't want people to know how picky I was, how uncomfortable I was with my Vietnamese-ness. But there I was, outed as a total asshole Vietnamese kid to all sorts of people, their eyes glaring at me, judging me in silence for my limited Americanized diet! I say "almost" ashamed, because the shame lasted I think until about dinnertime—when I ate another hamburger.

Don't get me wrong; I did eat some Vietnamese food. But I wasn't ready and didn't understand or appreciate Vietnamese food. That would take many more years and many, many more meals.

I do remember one early Vietnamese meal, though. That one time my parents took me to an underground restaurant in the Dallas suburb of Richardson, Texas. Now, this wasn't a rite of passage for every Vietnamese kid or something my trendy aviator glasses–wearing parents sought out as the latest craze in food. The restaurant was just another restaurant to them, the kind they used to eat at in Vietnam. Of course, you had to be in the know (high-five to my parents for being so cool), and in this case, a couple hundred people who didn't know me, my parents, or even cared to know us were in the know and crowded alongside us into a nondescript house in a random subdivision outside of the city limits. (If you offered me $1 million right now, I wouldn't be able to find the house, or even the neighborhood.)

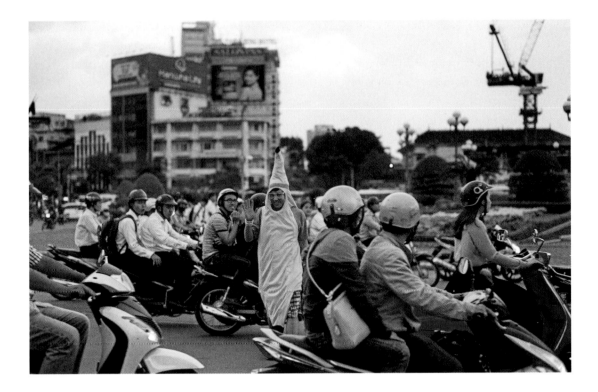

From the street, the house looked like, well, a house. Inside, though, it took on the atmosphere of a chaotic but fully functioning restaurant. It sure as hell wasn't a potluck, which in hindsight I probably should have thought was strange because, like I said, if you're Asian, you NEVER arrive at someone else's house without something edible in hand. I can't remember exactly what I ate. I can't remember how long we were there. I can't remember whether I was a punk, whether I cried and demanded KFC instead. I just remember that I took it all in, put one-and-one together, and figured out that even though this was not normal and it was potentially *illegal,* I really LIKED it—the energy, the feeling, the excitement of it all.

When I turned eighteen, my parents, most likely fed up with my white-washed American tendencies, decided it was time for me to visit Vietnam. It was finally time for me to "go back" to where it had all started for them, to visit the family I had always heard about but never had a connection with because they were a whole ocean and hemisphere away from me.

I'm not sure what I was thinking or expecting, but I can tell you, whatever it was, nothing played out the way I thought. First thing after landing in Saigon, my parents had to bribe the customs agent because I GUESS we looked like we had some money (FYI—back then the airport was not nearly as evolved and modern as it is now so that practice is not even close to as rampant today as it was twenty years ago).

My mom slipped the agent some cash and off we went into the heart of Saigon aka Ho Chi Minh City aka HCMC, which, FYI, every Vietnamese still calls Saigon.

And then we began our not-long-enough Christmas Vacation trip to meet family, and I got to put into practice all the elder-respecting lessons I'd been taught throughout my life. I saw and did things I'd never experienced before. My six-year-old cousin taught me how to properly cross Saigon streets (rule: you *go* and you *don't stop*). I hung out with my cousins of a similar age, my aunts, my uncles, and many other relatives who consistently commented on how cute I was. At this point I wasn't very comfortable with my looks so I thought they were being nice, a running theme of my life—being put on a pedestal, or not, based on looks alone—it's really astounding.

I finally got it . . . some of it . . . all of it. Who I was. What all this teaching was about. What my parents were about. And, for the first time, I felt connected to (and, conversely, realized how disconnected from it I had been) people who had faces, hair, skin color, and most everything else similar to mine . . . except I had been born in the United States.

To my surprise, and to my parent's delight, I even tried new food. The funny thing is that everything seemed to come together in my mom's hometown, where I ate one of the most delicious meals of my life. After spending time with extended family in Saigon, we hopped on a bus to Long Xuyen, my mom's hometown, where people speak a different dialect than in the North and South where most of her siblings and my grandmother still live to this day. My mom's oldest sisters operate a thriving sandal shop, inside a shophouse where they also live above. On one hot and muggy afternoon, my aunts got us *ca kho to,* caramelized catfish served in a claypot. It came with rendered and seemingly melted-on chunks of pork belly lining the sides of the claypot, which was also covered in the same delicious caramelized sauce that coated the catfish. Hesitantly, I ate it. The combination of the pork belly and catfish in my mouth made me immediately think, *Holy FUUUUUUUUUUUUUUUCK, I'm Vietnamese!* This was the food of my people, and I was PROUD to be Vietnamese.

Everything changed. Everything. The rules. My mind. The world. My palate. My respect for Vietnamese culture and food. Even my maturity. It's kind of like playing a Japanese role-playing game (JRPG for nerds like you and me) like *Final Fantasy,* which I played a lot of, when you get enough experience points to move to the next level of strength and intelligence and the fanfare music plays. That's what was going on through my soul when I ate that *ca kho to*. I leveled up. I grew up. A whole world of stuff that I had ignored was ahead of me, and then I knew that I wasn't just Vietnamese, I wasn't just American. I had achieved a new skill: the multi-hyphenated balance of being Vietnamese-fucking-American.

> Everything changed. Everything. The rules. My mind. The world. My palate. My respect for Vietnamese culture and food.

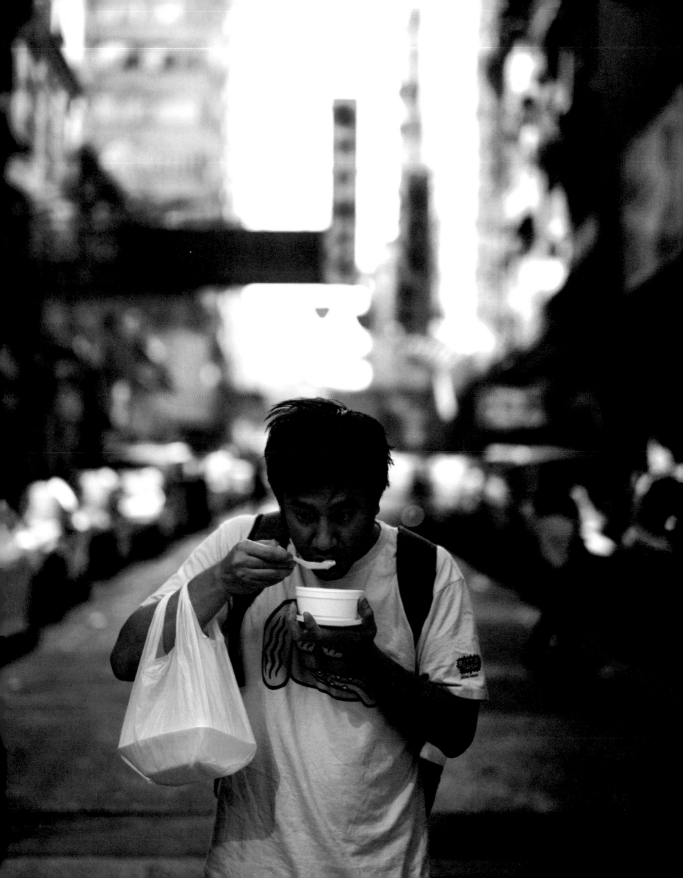

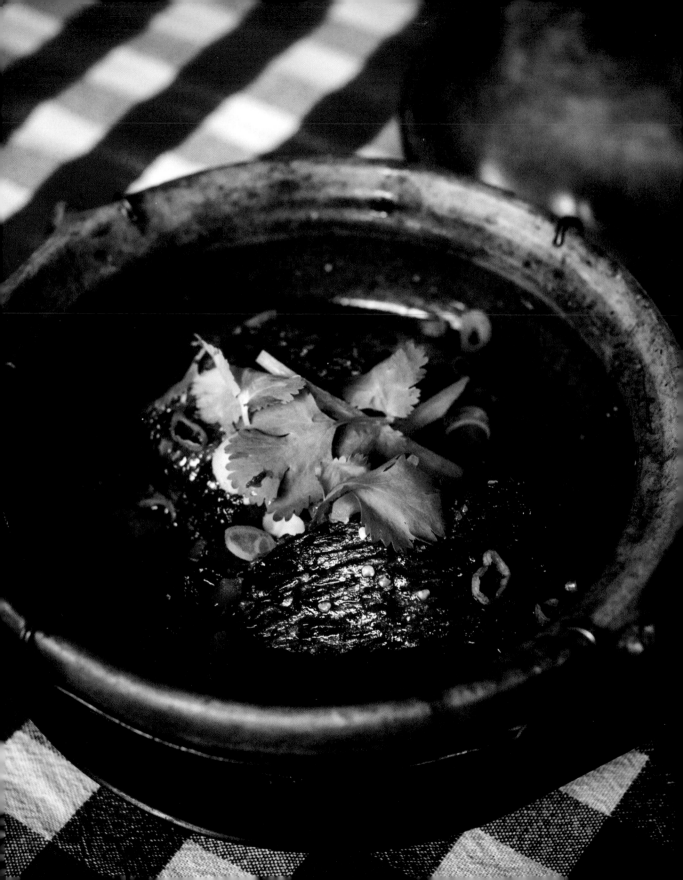

CLAYPOT CARAMELIZED STRIPED BASS

This is my favoritest dish in the entire universe (aka my "death row dish")! This is a classic Vietnamese dish, reimagined with Chinese-Vietnamese elements and made with a different marinated fish, grilled, then roasted with pancetta—all amazingly delicious in your mouth. Typically served with rice or Roast Pork Belly XO Fried Rice for the super flavor winning combo.

2–4 SERVINGS

1½ pounds fresh striped bass, scaled and cut into 1½ inch steaks

6 tablespoons fish sauce

4½ tablespoons firmly packed brown sugar

3 tablespoons plus 1 tablespoon minced shallots

3 tablespoons minced garlic

1 teaspoon coarsely ground black pepper

6 pancetta cubes (¾-inch)

1 tablespoon Caramel Sauce (page 239)

1 tablespoon minced ginger

1 Thai chili, sliced*

1½ cups young coconut juice†

1 pinch kosher salt

GARNISHES:

1 pinch coarsely ground black pepper

1 tablespoon chopped scallions

2 stalks cilantro, hand ripped

6 slices Fresno chilies

* Do not rub your eyes after slicing these bad boys!

† Preferably from a fresh young coconut. It makes a huge difference.

BALLS OUT
40–80 SERVINGS

30 pounds fresh striped bass, scaled and cut into 1½ inch steaks

7⅓ cups tablespoons fish sauce

5½ cups firmly packed brown sugar

3⅔ cups plus 1¼ cups minced shallots

3⅔ cups minced garlic

6⅔ tablespoons coarsely ground black pepper

120 pancetta cubes (¾-inch)

1¼ cups Caramel Sauce (page 239)

1¼ cups minced ginger

20 Thai chilies, sliced*

7½ quarts young coconut juice†

1¼ teaspoons kosher salt

GARNISHES:

1¼ teaspoons coarsely ground black pepper

1¼ cups chopped scallions

40 stalks cilantro, ripped

120 slices Fresno chilies

1. Preheat oven to 450°F. Clean fish steaks, rinse well, and pat dry.
2. Combine fish sauce, brown sugar, shallots, garlic, and pepper in a mixing bowl. Mix until sugar dissolves. Coat fish with fish sauce mix and marinate for 30 minutes on each side (60 minutes total). Do not marinate any longer than this, because the fish will get too salty.
3. Remove fish from marinade and shake off excess. Set aside.
4. Next, sauté and brown pancetta in a pan with a little bit of cooking oil over high heat. Set aside.
5. In the same pan, sear fish with some cooking oil over medium-high heat until fish turns a nice golden color that you would actually consider paying money for at a nice restaurant like Starry Kitchen. Transfer fish into a claypot (or a cast iron skillet or oven-safe pan you can cover), and add pancetta. Set aside.
6. Then pour Caramel Sauce evenly over fish and let it sit.
7. In the same pan in which you seared the fish, add ginger, the remaining shallots, and Thai chili and sauté over medium-high heat for 10–15 seconds, or until brown. Add coconut juice and a pinch of salt while deglazing the pan over high heat, scraping and stirring in all the delicious bits of flavor (aka "the fond"). Once the sauce comes to a boil, immediately pour over fish.
8. Cover the claypot, place on the middle rack in the oven, and bake for 7–8 minutes, or until fish temperature reaches 140°F or higher.

Remove from oven, garnish with coarse black pepper, scallions, cilantro, and Fresno chilies. Prepare for the afterlife because now you can die in complete and utter sated peace and happiness.

Fresh fish is always best. If you're picking up one on ice or refrigerated, be sure to check its eyes, which should be clear. If they are cloudy, with a stoned/ glazed-over look, the fish has been dead for quite a while. Try to find a fresher fish with clearer eyes.

Ask the (Asian store) fishmonger to scale your fish and slice it into 1½-inch-thick steaks. (If you own a fish scaler, or you're OCD like us, you'll probably want to re-scale it at home because even the best fishmongers get distracted.) If you're shopping for fish at a Whole *cough* Paycheck *cough cough* market, they conveniently cut them for you but charge way more than the current average price of $6 per pound. #justsayin

GRILLED FISH HEADS AND TAILS

When you own a restaurant, you use lots of fresh ingredients and you're almost always broke (ain't no joke), so you want to make sure everything you spend is worth it—and you can never, never, never let ANYTHING go to waste. We buy fresh whole fish for the Claypot Caramelized Striped Bass, but that recipe doesn't include fish heads and fish tails. So to make them useful (and us less broke), we grill the heads and fry the tails, which is deliciously simple, especially served with Vietnamese fish sauce and whichever pickled vegetable strikes your fancy.

BALLS OUT
40–80 SERVINGS

4 cups vegetable or canola oil

32 bunches scallions, chopped

2 teaspoons kosher salt

20 fish heads

20 fish tails

Ground black pepper, for seasoning

2½ cups all-purpose flour

2½ cups cornstarch

Mushroom bouillon, to taste

Scallions, chopped, for garnish

2–4 SERVINGS

2 tablespoons vegetable or canola oil

1 bunch scallions, chopped

1 pinch Kosher salt

1 fish head

1 fish tail

Ground black pepper, for seasoning

2 tablespoons all-purpose flour

2 tablespoons cornstarch

Mushroom bouillon, to taste

Scallions, chopped, for garnish

Coco Rico Vietnamese Fish Sauce (page 240; optional)

1. Bring a pan to medium-high heat. Add oil, scallions, and salt, then mix. When scallions wilt, your oil is done. Remove from heat, set aside. Store in a container and refrigerate.
2. You can grill or fry your heads and tails (we prefer to grill the head, and fry the tail). Grilling is a great option because heads are often too big to fry, and a nice char from the grill really brings out the flavor of the fish, particularly its cheeks, which in my opinion (and most of Asia's, as I've been told) is the best part of the fish.
3. If you're frying just the tail, heat 1 inch oil in a small pot over medium-high heat to 350°F. If you aren't able to use a barbecue grill or oven broiler, increase the oil to at least 2 inches to make room for that head.
4. Clean the fish head and tail under cold water until there is no visible blood coming from the head. Make sure to remove the gills if there are any. Pat dry.

5. If you're grilling, turn the grill up to medium-high heat. Brush both sides of the fish head with cooking oil. Salt and pepper like you see in slow motion in all those fancy cooking shows and make it rain. Massage in salt and pepper, inside and out. Grill that head for about 5–7 minutes. Don't turn over until the head can be lifted relatively cleanly without losing much amazingly delicious skin in the process.

6. If frying heads and tails, double up on both flour and cornstarch in the next step.

7. Combine flour and cornstarch in a bowl. Season with salt, pepper, and mushroom bouillon and mix. Taste the flour mixture and adjust seasoning.

   In mixing bowl, coat fish tails (and fish head), if you're not grilling it, in flour/cornstarch mixture. When the pot of oil is ready, fry coated fish parts for about 5–7 minutes until golden brown, turning frequently. Remove, shake off excess oil, and plate. Drizzle on 1 tablespoon scallion oil and garnish with scallions and a side of Coco Rico Fish Sauce for dipping.

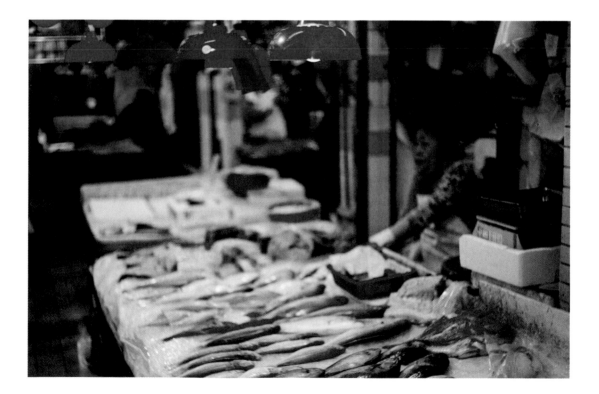

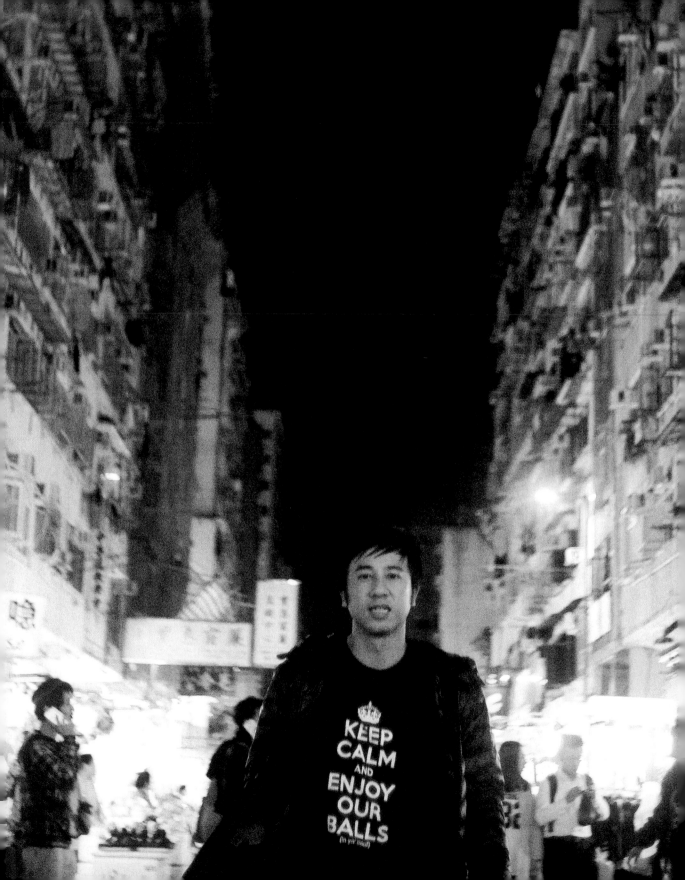

SECOND POP-UP/ BUTTON MASH

LEGAL *LOOPHOLES* AND WHY I KEEP *GETTING INTO* AND *OUT OF* TROUBLE

LET'S INTRODUCE A NEW PLAYER INTO THE LINEUP OF THE CRAZY PEOPLE WHO MAKE UP THE LIVES OF ME AND THI. **PLEASE MEET MOHAMMED "MO" BUTTS KASHMIRI.** MO IS AN AS-LIBERAL-AS-THEY-COME PAKISTANI-AMERICAN (THERE'S THAT DIASPORIC MULTI-HYPHENATE FOR ANYONE FOLLOWING ALONG!) WITH A THICK-AS-TEXAS-TOAST ACCENT, AND HE WAS ONE OF MY CLOSEST FRIENDS IN COLLEGE.

He was also my partner in crime for many a hell-raising and someone who helped me coin the phrase "celebrating our failure"—which basically means recognizing failures being just as important as recognizing successes—by getting drunk over many (or one if you're me) Mi Cocina margaritas. Rather than cry about something, Mo and I both believed you should revel in it, because at the very least there's always a good story to tell—and an excuse to get drunk, too! If he's not the most important player in the story of my life, he's definitely one of the most important, the catalyst who brought out the hell-raiser in me, the kind of fearless, balls-out adventurer I always wanted

to be but for whatever reason couldn't fully tap into. Though he continues to raise hell as a professional union organizer, Mo would tell you I've taken his guidance too far since our freshman year at UT Dallas.

I first met Mo in chemistry class, when he and I were still pre-med. He astounded me. He showed up to class, never took notes, always killed during discussions, and carried himself with a swagger that was different from anyone else. Most people came in and out of the class-room with a little bit of fear. But Mo walked around without a care (or fear) in the world. This unlikely confidence stems from the fact that he has what nerdy science-like people call a "photographic memory." He was the hilarious lil' Pakistani-American guy who packed a whole lot of fucking punch.

I started hanging out with him during my junior year, right around the same time I was considering joining the Student Government Association (SGA). I should include here that my heavily conservative coinstigator, Matt Grygar, persuaded me to run for Vice President of SGA shortly after I joined. Without a doubt, Matt is the most conservative friend Thi and I have. He's super Catholic, and if you looked up a picture of a shit-kicker, his handsomely ugly mug might proudly appear there too. I guess I have him to blame, along with Mo, for feeding my addiction to power, winning, and . . . just fucking shit up!

When I was running for a position on SGA, Mo was vice president and another friend (and former hair model), Kim Caylor, was president. In addition to my love of getting involved and helping people, I also really love working with people I like, regardless of the cause or activity. Because Mo and Kim were already involved with SGA, it seemed like the most natural thing for me to get all extracurricular and be part of something again. This was an important and pivotal time in my life.

We organized events to inform the student body of changes happening on campus and tell them about rights they didn't know they had, and, in the early days of the Internet, instituted an online voting system. But the most important event in the crossing of Mo and me involved an online teacher evaluation system.

We wanted a way for students to avoid total assholes when signing up for classes, and Yelp hadn't been invented yet, and the Internet as a forum for the mainstream to share their opinions (aka trolling) wasn't really legitimate yet. We figured that students already evaluated professors verbally when they asked friends about this or that professor and how hard he/she was and whether he/she was a total jerk. Our idea was to create a much larger database that students could use as a central resource. In hindsight, I also would have told professors that they would have a chance to see what students were saying about them and their curriculum and, in the process, learn how to improve on the negatives that they might agree with. But we weren't mature enough to think that far ahead, and anyway, disrupting things, or "fucking shit up," was really our life motto at the time.

So we set up the forum, started testing it out—and then the university immediately put the kibosh on it. The university was concerned about students who passionately hated their professors enough to potentially write false statements about their professors, which legally could be deemed as libelous or defaming a professor's character. We knew this was a real concern. But giving up so easily went against why we were doing this in the first place. To stand firm, we chose to instead ignore this "conversation" and proceed with the plan. Because, really, what could the university do to us?

Well, we found out exactly what the University of Texas (UT) System, backed by the State of Texas, could do. They sent us a cease-and-desist letter. But under Mo's guidance, we still ignored it. And then things got really funny! We were invited to a video teleconference call with the General Counsel of the UT System, which is a fancy way of saying, the entire fucking legal team for the entire state-wide UT System.

Now THAT was intimidating. What's helpful to note is that Mo changed course (like most college students) early on in our undergraduate careers from pre-med and started down the path of law school and politics. He was great at it, and inspired that side of me, too, such that I ALMOST took the LSAT because I aspired to be in politics (and for fun, because it has a logic games section. I still wanna take it, dammit!). I also started moving down that path because I DO love working a room, working with people, and affecting change. With all that said, Mo had more of a plan than I knew at the time. But he divulged the details to me only right before we went into the meeting.

We were in a special room in the computer science building, the most high-tech of all the buildings on campus—in the prehistoric days before Skype—with a badass video teleconference system. As the lights dimmed and a video screen came down out of the ceiling, about twelve, yeah TWELVE, attorneys appeared onscreen and one began talking to us about libel and defamation of character and whether we understood what it all meant—like we were in third grade! They might as well have fed us Jell-O with whipped cream, patted us on the heads, and sent us off to recess. It was pretty condescending and almost demoralizing.

At the end of the jibba-jabba legal talk, we were told that if we continued on the path we

And this was the event that set me down an eighteen-year-long path to continually fuck shit up and find a simple solution in every problem.

〜〜〜

were pursuing, the state—the HUGE state of motherfucking Texas, Tejas, home of the Alamo, Sam Houston, and all his debauchery, the Lone Star, and "The stars at night, are big and bright (*clap clap clap clap*) *Deep in the Heart of Texaaaaaaaaaaaaas!*", this state, our great state that houses Whataburger, Dairy Queen (the "Texas Stop Sign," ya know), and motherfucking tasty Tex-Mex, *that* state—was going to "take action" . . . they were going to SUE US!

I'll admit, that statement made my heart stop pretty quickly. But this is where Mo dropped the bomb and David-and-Goliath'ed them across the dedicated ISDN (prefiber, for all you techies out there) from Dallas to Austin and knocked them—with their six-figure salaries, fancy cars, fancy degrees from prestigious law schools, trophy spouses, and privileged kids in hard-to-get-into private schools—back into their cushy seats with a few choice words . . .

"Sue us? For what, money? We're college students. *We don't have any MONEY!*"

And then we both laughed (him confidently, me nervously at first, and then the reality struck toward full-hilarity manic-speed laughing) like kids hocked up on laughing gas in a dentist's office at the notion because there is only one reason to sue anyone—for money, which we clearly didn't have as I was living on instant ramen, peanut butter and jelly sandwiches, and the sometimes weekly Costco run of artificially preserved chicken that my mom would drop off. Thanks, Mom!

An uncomfortable silence fell on the administrators in the room with us and, most definitely, on the Austin crowd as well. Remember those Sprint commercials where they dropped a pin to show how clearly your loved ones would come through over their phone lines? It was exactly that quiet, but the feeling was like a thousand pins had fallen to literally deafen them at the ridicule that they would receive if they sued broke-ass students.

It was clearly a win on our side. I couldn't believe it. I had no experience in this kind of thing—litigation, law studies—none of it. And the simple logic of it was pristine, clean, and motherfucking mean. It's like we were playing chess, and you could feel the call of "checkmate" from our side.

I don't remember the Office of General Counsel saying much after that other than just ending the conversation immediately. The screen disappeared back up into the ceiling, the projector was turned off, and the lights were raised, as if the greatest movie of a lifetime was over. I looked at Mo in amazement.

Most people look up to sports figures or historical leaders, but at that moment, I looked up to that little Pakistani-American friend of mine, even though he was shorter than me so I actually looked down on him. And this was the event that set me down an eighteen-year-long path to continually fuck shit up and find a simple solution in every problem.

Oh, one final anecdote. Mo later sued the University of California (UC) System on behalf of the entire UC student body, winning a temporary injunction of $40 million for the students over the issue of fee increases during a crazy California financial crisis that got the current governor, Gray Davis, impeached and opened the door for the next (Terminator) governor, Arnold Schwarzenegger, to come in. I protested with him at one of the meetings of the UC Board of Regents because I really missed hell-raising. Like I mentioned in the introduction, during the protest, we were almost busted by the cops for selling T-shirts—until we pointed out that we were just taking donations: the shirts were free. This loophole stuck with me for a long time and was what I specifically applied in the inception of Starry Kitchen. I exploited this loophole whenever we got busted. And I always got away with it.

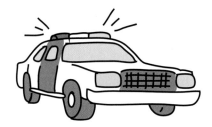

SODA CHANH (AKA VIETNAMESE LIME SODA)

This is such a refreshing drink, and a great base if you want to make a version of a mojito or add some vodka for a tasty recreational beverage. But you don't have to . . . unless you LOVE alcohol—then go right on ahead.

BALLS OUT
40–80 SERVINGS

DOUBLE-CONCENTRATED SIMPLE SYRUP:

5 quarts water

10 quarts sugar

SODA CHANH:

160 large limes, halved*

20 liters club soda or sparkling water or tonic water

2–4 SERVINGS

DOUBLE-CONCENTRATED SIMPLE SYRUP:

1 cup water

2 cups sugar

SODA CHANH:

8 large limes, halved*

1 liter club soda or sparkling water or tonic water (which ARE different and will slightly affect the flavor because of the differing salt content)

Double-Concentrated Simple Syrup

Mint leaves

* The type of lime you use changes how delicious this drink is, but any kind of lime, like calamansi limes or key limes, works well. Oh, and if you use small limes, definitely double the lime count.

1. **FOR THE "SHUGA" (AKA SIMPLE SYRUP):** Bring a pot with water and sugar to medium heat, stirring constantly until sugar completely dissolves in water. Remove simple syrup from heat, let cool, and transfer to a container. Store covered in the refrigerator when not in use.

2. **FOR SODA CHANH:** Fill four tall 12-fluid-ounce glasses up with ice cubes. Then fill each glass three-quarters of the way to the top with club soda.

3. Next, squeeze four lime halves by hand into each glass. (Or if you have a fancy juicer, have at it with your new-fangled technology; it'll work, too, but you won't get that tactile satisfaction or the show of squeezing them by hand. You also won't get that burning sensation if you have any cuts whatsoever on your hand.)

4. Add 4–6 tablespoons simple syrup to each glass. Different types of limes will change the appropriate balance of required sweetness. Stir well. And just like with food, TASTE IT. It should taste a tad sweet, a tad tart, but not so stringent on your palette. Add more at your sugary leisure.

And now you can be like a hipster bartender, take some mint leaves, and slap 'em into the palm of your hand (which brings out the aroma really well by the way—that's not just a fancy pencil-thin-mustache-wearing hipster move). Throw a couple of leaves on top of each drink. Top off with a little more of your carbonated liquid beverage, stir to get some of the mint aroma into your glass, garnish with one more hand-clapped mint leaf, and serve either with a deep Southern accent or cursing like a Vietnamese coffee shop patron—and enjoy!

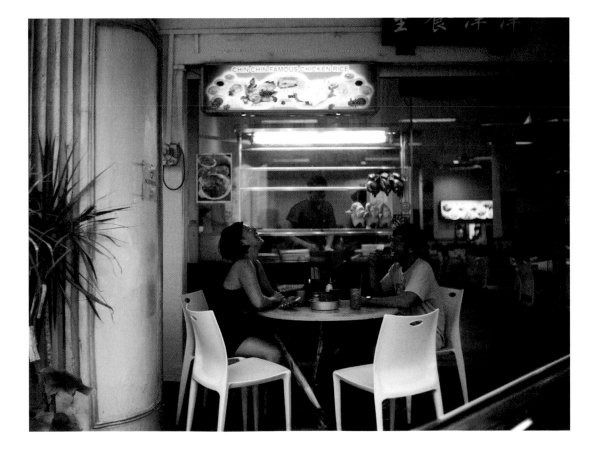

WATERMELON GINGER AGUA FRESCA

Sweet and spiced drinktasticness. Keep it chilled, and keep chill y'all.

BALLS OUT
40-80 SERVINGS

10 slices (30 ounces) ginger

5 cups Double-Concentrated Simple Syrup*

60 pounds (about 15 quarts) fresh seedless watermelon†

15 cups cold water

---

1 slice (3 ounces) ginger

½ cup Double-Concentrated Simple Syrup (refer to Soda Chanh for recipe)*

6 pounds (about 6 cups) fresh seedless watermelon†

1½ cups cold water

* Ginger liquor is a nice replacement if you want to go a lil boozy with this.

† Don't chuck those rinds, though! Make some Pickled Watermelon Rinds!

1. Crush the ginger with the flat side of a cleaver or a heavy object. Add ginger and simple syrup to a pot, bring to a simmer over low heat. Once it simmers, remove from heat and allow it to sit for at least 10 minutes so the ginger completely infuses the syrup.
2. Cut open a watermelon, cut the "flesh" off of the rinds, set aside rinds for some amazing pickling, cut the flesh into small enough pieces to fit in your blender. Puree away. If the consistency isn't quite liquid yet, mix in water and blend again. If you have seeds, blend away anyway. They will be filtered out in the next step.
3. Pour the watermelon puree through a chinois or fine mesh sieve into a pitcher. Repeat the puree process with more watermelon flesh until you get 6–7 cups worth of puree.
4. From the top of the juice in the pitcher, skim off foam and dispose.
5. Add remaining water (if any), and 7½ teaspoons of your recently infused ginger simple syrup. Mix in, taste, and add more ginger syrup to your liking (don't worry, I made double what we recommend for all you sugary drink lovers out there).

    Stir before serving. Fill glasses with ice cubes, pour Agua Fresca over them, and chug away. Many an exciting watermelon escapade awaits you. (I *really* like watermelon!)

GINGER SESAME RAINBOW ROASTED CARROTS (AKA ROASTED CARROTS WITH SWEET SOY GLAZE)

Like most American kids, I grew up mainly on canned vegetables and common vegetables available at the most common grocery stores. A lot later in life, though, I found out that vegetables don't necessarily taste like . . . what they *should* taste like. "Heirloom" vegetables are supposed to be the original versions before they were mangled/modified/evolved into something completely different. And now I understand why I hated vegetables so much as a kid. But really, holy SHIT BALLS, BATMAN! Real vegetables are really good!

BALLS OUT
40–80 SERVINGS

FOR THE SWEET SOY GLAZE:

5 cups honey

5 cups light soy sauce

1¼ cups dark brown sugar

6⅔ tablespoons minced garlic

3⅓ tablespoons finely grated fresh ginger

1⅔ tablespoons crushed red pepper flakes

FOR THE CARROTS:

120 whole (about 6¼ pounds) multicolored rainbow carrots

1¼ cups butter (optional)*

2½ cups sweet soy glaze

2–4 SERVINGS

FOR THE SWEET SOY GLAZE:

¼ cup honey

¼ cup light soy sauce

1 tablespoon dark brown sugar

1 teaspoon minced garlic

½ teaspoon finely grated fresh ginger

¼ teaspoon crushed red pepper flakes

FOR THE CARROTS:

6 whole (about 5 ounces) multicolored rainbow carrots

1 tablespoon butter (optional)*

2 tablespoons sweet soy glaze

* Use the butter if you aren't grilling. Oh, but you know what's even better . . . CLARIFIED BUTTER MOTHERF**ERS!

1. Combine glaze ingredients and vigorously marry them all together. DO IT!
2. If you have a grill, grilling will bring out the flavor in the carrots best. Set it to a medium-high flame. If you don't have a grill, sauté carrots in a pan with butter on medium-high to high heat.
3. Cook until they're blistered, nice and golden. Add in the glaze (or brush on the glaze if you're grilling), toss carrots in sauce, then remove from heat, cool 'em down, remove from the pan, and halve vertically.

   Plate any fancy way you want. And then eat them (including the stems which are super tasty), destroying all the fancy plating you just put your time and effort into.

MISO CHARRED BRUSSELS SPROUTS

I'm pretty sure that after creating this dish, the Spam Brussels Sprout Fried Rice came into being because we wanted another way to use Brussels. Or maybe the other way around. In my humble opinion, the best way to run a kitchen is to find multiple and equally delicious uses for your ingredients and thus . . . this dish (or the fried rice) was invented and owes its existence to fried rice (or this dish). Either way, time to bow down to Brussels!

BALLS OUT

40–80 SERVINGS

FOR CHILI MISO SAUCE:

2¾ cups sugar

2½ tablespoons white miso

3¼ cups light soy sauce

7½ tablespoons rice vinegar

10 tablespoons sake

7½ tablespoons chili garlic sauce

BRUSSELS:

10 pounds Brussels sprouts, halved

10 tablespoons butter

2½ cups Chili Miso Sauce

Kosher salt and pepper

2–4 SERVINGS

FOR CHILI MISO SAUCE:

3 tablespoons sugar

½ teaspoon white miso

3½ tablespoons light soy sauce

½ tablespoon rice vinegar

2 teaspoons sake

½ tablespoon chili garlic sauce

BRUSSELS:

½ pound Brussels sprouts, halved

½ tablespoon butter (and even better than clarified butter . . . BROWN butter)

4 tablespoons Chili Miso Sauce

Kosher salt and pepper

1. Dissolve sugar in white miso and soy sauce in a pan over low heat. Next, add rice vinegar, sake, and chili garlic sauce. Mix it well. Remove from heat and set aside.

2. Toss Brussels sprouts with a little bit of oil in a bowl; lightly salt and pepper while tossing.

3. Bring a pan up to high heat and add butter and Brussels sprouts once the pan is hot. Sauté 2–3 minutes until you get a nice even and crispy char across all the Brussels. If the Brussels are a tad dry, splash some water to rehydrate them. Next, add Chili Miso Sauce and stir-fry for another minute, making sure Brussels are fully coated in sauce. Remove from heat, plate, and get in there!

MUSTARD GREENS AND PANCETTA

Sometimes the simplest dishes are the most delicious. Oh, and this dish goes to show you that not all vegetable dishes have to be healthy (because, beef fat) or plainly vegetarian (because, pancetta).

BALLS OUT

40–80 SERVINGS

18 pounds young Chinese mustard greens

1¼ cups Beef Tallow/ Rendered Beef Fat (page 238) or cooking oil

5 pounds pancetta, cut into ½-inch to ¾-inch cubes

140 garlic cloves, crushed

10 tablespoons mushroom bouillon

3⅓ tablespoons palm sugar

80 whole Thai chilies, dry roasted until lightly brown

2–4 SERVINGS

14½ ounces young Chinese mustard greens

1 tablespoon Beef Tallow/Rendered Beef Fat (page 238) or cooking oil

4 ounces pancetta, cut into ½-inch to ¾-inch cubes

7 garlic cloves, crushed

½ tablespoon mushroom bouillon

½ teaspoon palm sugar

4 whole Thai chilies, dry roasted until lightly brown

1. Tear mustard green leaves off of the bunch. If the stem/root is too thick, cut it off and dispose. Clean the leaves thoroughly.

    OPTIONAL: To make the greens a tad less bitter, massage them with salt, then wash the salt off. We personally love the bitterness, but the bitter flavor can be overpowering for some people.

2. Slice each leaf in half down the middle, lengthwise. Fold cut halves over each other and cut (widthwise) the leafy parts into 2-inch sections. Cut stem parts about 1 inch wide.

3. Heat pan on high heat. Once the pan is hot, add ½ tablespoon Beef Tallow and sauté pancetta. Once browned, remove pancetta from heat. Set aside.

    Add remaining Beef Tallow and sauté garlic. Next, add mustard greens and stir-fry until the leafy greens shrink. Decrease to medium heat and add mushroom bouillon and sugar and hand break the whole dried chili into pieces into the pan. Toss pancetta back in, stir-fry, then remove from heat, plate, serve family-style with rice, and convert people to the dark fatty beef side of preparing vegetables.

CANTO-STYLE CHAYOTE, ENOKI, AND GOJI BERRIES

Chayote is a special vegetable/fruit/gourd, not unlike squash. It's not very pretty, but it's pretty cheap, and it has a great crunch and takes flavors surprisingly well.

BALLS OUT
40–80 SERVINGS

2½ cups goji berries

40 chayote, julienned

20 (5.3-ounce) packs enoki mushrooms, roots cut off

100 cloves garlic, crushed

1¼ cups Chinese cooking wine

10 tablespoons veggie stir-fry sauce

3⅓ tablespoons palm sugar

5 tablespoons mushroom bouillon

2–4 SERVINGS

1 heaping tablespoon goji berries

2 chayote, julienned

1 (5.3-ounce) pack enoki mushrooms, roots cut off

5 cloves garlic, crushed

1 tablespoon Chinese cooking wine

1½ teaspoon Lee Kum Kee brand veggie stir-fry sauce*

½ teaspoon palm sugar

¾ teaspoon mushroom bouillon

* This sauce is made up of all sorts of vegetarian umami-ness, and is kind of like a mixture of oyster sauce and a mushroom sauce . . . but with no fish or meat ingredients. Vegetarians should check this shit out!

1. Soak goji berries in a bowl of water until soft. Set aside.
2. In order to cut chayote properly, first halve it. Slice halves evenly between ¼- to ½-inch thick, then julienne slices into evenly square-tipped strips. Dispose of any strips with the core and seeds.
3. Tear enoki mushrooms into small bunches and strands. Set aside in a separate bowl.
4. Once goji berries are soft, drain bowl completely. Keep goji berries in bowl.
5. In a pan, sauté garlic with some cooking oil over high heat until light brown and fragrant. Next, add chayote. Stir-fry and sear for 30 seconds. Add cooking wine and sauté for another 20–30 seconds.
6. Next, mix in veggie stir-fry sauce, palm sugar, and mushroom bouillon and sauté for 5–10 seconds; then add goji berries and enoki mushrooms and stir-fry for another 5–10 seconds.

    When chayote is between crunchy and slightly soft, remove from heat, plate, and garnish with freshly cracked black pepper. Serve.

SHRIMP TOAST (BRUSCHETTA)

What can I say about shrimp toast other than . . . SHRIMP TOOOOAAAAAST! And it's not really much of a bruschetta, except for the nice refreshing tomato on a buttery shrimp paste on toast. But ya know what, it's good with that slice of toast and tomato.☺ Oh, make sure the bread's strong enough to hold up a hefty and dense layer o' shrimp. If it's too soft (like delicious Wonder bread), it'll break apart, you'll be sad, and you'll hate us for forever.☺

BALLS OUT
40–80 SERVINGS

5 pounds (any size) shrimp, thawed, peeled, and deveined

2½ cups plus 2½ teaspoons kosher salt

2½ cups plus 1⅔ tablespoons cornstarch or tapioca starch

2½ teaspoons sugar

3⅓ tablespoons chicken bouillon

1¼ teaspoons black pepper

6⅔ tablespoons minced garlic

20 stalks scallion, minced

6⅔ tablespoons minced ginger

2½ ounces cilantro

1¼ cups (~10 large eggs) egg white

2½ teaspoons water

5 tablespoons cooking oil

60 slices white bread

2–4 SERVINGS

½ pound (any size) shrimp, thawed, peeled, and deveined

¼ cup plus ¼ teaspoon kosher salt

¼ cup plus ½ teaspoon cornstarch or tapioca starch

¼ teaspoon sugar

1 teaspoon chicken bouillon

2 pinches black pepper

2 teaspoons minced garlic

2 stalks scallion, minced

2 teaspoons minced ginger

¼ ounce cilantro

2 tablespoons (~1 large egg) egg white

¼ teaspoon water

½ tablespoon cooking oil

6 slices white bread

Tomatoes, thinly sliced, for garnish

Cilantro, coarsely chopped, for garnish

1. Toss shrimp in a colander with ¼ cup salt and ¼ cup cornstarch. Massage shrimp, then rinse immediately under cold water. Gently squeeze to wring out excess water, pat dry, and transfer to a bowl.
2. Combine remaining cornstarch and salt with sugar, chicken bouillon, and black pepper in a separate bowl. Mix well, then toss with shrimp.
3. Drop that same shrimp in a food processor and sporadically pulse until mixture is between coarsely chopped and fine. Do not puree; that's taking things waaay too far, kids. Remove and set aside in a bowl.
4. Next, add garlic, scallions, ginger, cilantro, egg whites, water, and oil. Mix well, using your hands until completely mixed in. Cover and refrigerate for 1 hour.
5. Once you're good and ready, remove the shrimp "spread" from the fridge and spread evenly (<-key word) on a nice piece o' bread. Don't get heavy handed in the middle of the bread; everyone spreads it too

thick in the middle, which prevents the spread from cooking evenly all around. Repeat until you have exhausted all of the shrimp spread.

6. Next, heat a pan with some oil on medium-high heat, sear the shrimp toast "spread" side down, cook through until evenly golden brown from edge to edge, then flip over to toast and crisp up the other side.

Plate and garnish with tomatoes, black pepper, and chopped cilantro, and cut into diagonal quarters for a nice appetizer or snack—the best shrimpy bruschetta of your life.

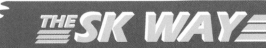

THE SK WAY

Even if you get yourself peeled, head-off, and deveined shrimp, we still recommend taking a moment to inspect the shrimp for a black vein across the back. If it's there, use a knife to slit the back of the shrimp's body along the vein and handily remove that slippery black sucker out.

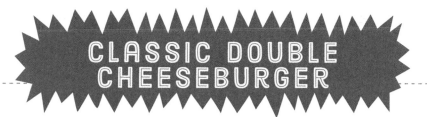
CLASSIC DOUBLE CHEESEBURGER

I have to give huge inspirational credit to Jordan Weiss, one of our Button Mash partners, for the simple suggestion of including a classic double cheeseburger on the menu . . . of an Asian restaurant bar arcade—which somehow makes sense to me! Taking a break from delicious Banh Mi sammies and switching to burgers ain't such a bad thing to do.☺

    We put about one year of research into our burger (food research is the best kind). The immediate influences: Whataburger (Texas FOREVER!); Bill & Hiroko's Burgers, local to us in Van Nuys; the old-school Belcampo Burger at Grand Central Market; and the most influential burger of all of them, Pie 'n Burger in Pasadena.

BALLS OUT
40–80 SERVINGS

Butter, melted or softened to room temperature

80 Bimbo hamburger buns

Kosher salt and pepper

40 pounds (160 patties) 80–20 ground Angus chuck, or a custom blend with leaner cuts, shaped into thin 5- to 6-inch-wide ¼ pound patties

160 slices American cheese or medium cheddar

Yellow mustard

Pickled Persian Cucumbers (page 248)

Red onion, sliced ⅛ to ¼ inch thick

Butter lettuce, cleaned and separated

Tomato, sliced ¼ inch thick

2–4 SERVINGS

Butter, melted or softened to room temperature

4 Bimbo hamburger buns, or a similarly "enriched" squishy burger bun (no brioche—don't do it!)

Kosher salt and pepper

2 pounds (8 patties) 80–20 ground Angus chuck or a custom blend

with leaner cuts, shaped into thin 5- to 6-inch-wide ¼-pound patties

8 slices American cheese or medium cheddar cheese (American cheese is classic; cheddar gives a different, beefier kind of burger)

Yellow mustard

Pickled Persian Cucumbers (page 248)

Red onion, sliced ⅛ to ¼ inch thick—thick enough to get that onion crunch with every bite!

Butter lettuce, cleaned and separated

Tomato, sliced ¼ inch thick—who needs ketchup when there's a tomato?

1. Heat a pan/griddle to medium-high heat. Spread top and bottom of buns with butter, lay open-face down in pan and cook for 1–2 minutes. Once the buns get a golden and almost crispy crust, remove from pan and set aside on a plate. In that same pan, add a tiny bit of cooking oil, and liberally sprinkle a layer of equal amounts of salt and pepper in the pan. Next, add beef patties and cook 3–4 minutes, while frequently smothering patties into pan. Don't move patties until they get a nicely browned salt-and-pepper crust.

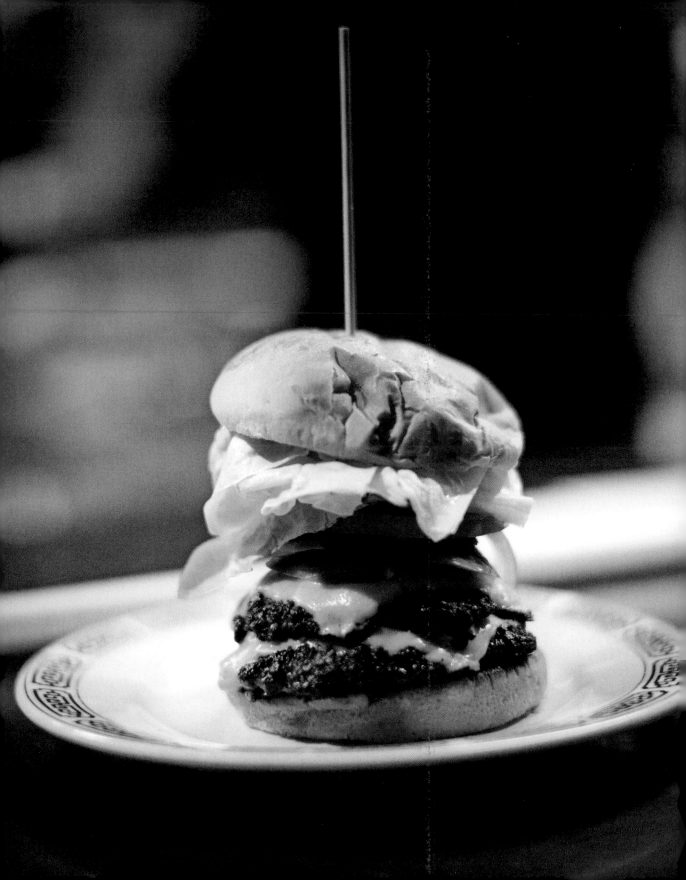

2. Once they're encrusted with those tasty crunchy burger bits, temporarily remove patties from pan. Add another layer of equal amounts salt and pepper to the pan, then flip the uncooked side of the patties down into the pan. Let the smothering continue.

3. Note: cook the burgers close to well done to achieve that awesome salt-and-pepper crunchy crust. (I know, BLASPHEMY!)

4. Add a slice of cheese on top of each patty while still in the pan.

5. As the cheese melts, spread a thin layer of mustard on the open-side of the bottom buns, remove and stack two patties on the bottom bun, then layer the burger with pickles, onions, tomato, lettuce, and the top bun.

With all ingredient powers combined, "the power is YOURS" to enjoy the spoils of our extensive burger research for maximum burger consumption and pleasure.

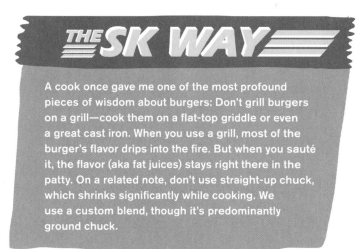

THE SK WAY

A cook once gave me one of the most profound pieces of wisdom about burgers: Don't grill burgers on a grill—cook them on a flat-top griddle or even a great cast iron. When you use a grill, most of the burger's flavor drips into the fire. But when you sauté it, the flavor (aka fat juices) stays right there in the patty. On a related note, don't use straight-up chuck, which shrinks significantly while cooking. We use a custom blend, though it's predominantly ground chuck.

ALMOND "TOFU" JELL-O

If you had given this dish to a younger me, I would not have appreciated how sweet it isn't. I would have been a jerk. I would have been dramatic. And I would have been . . . *wrong*. Now, I love how refreshing and balanced this dish is.

Aside from all that, this is actually a VEGAN dessert (if you don't serve it with evaporated milk), because we use agar-agar, a seaweed-based "gelatin." Yay!

BALLS OUT
40–80 SERVINGS

3 quarts cold water

3 cups sugar

8 cups unsweetened soy milk *

10 teaspoons almond extract

10 teaspoons agar-agar

5 cups evaporated milk

2–4 SERVINGS

1½ cups cold water

6 tablespoons sugar

1 cup unsweetened soy milk *

1¼ teaspoons almond extract

1¼ teaspoons agar-agar

½ cup evaporated milk

Fresh strawberries, thinly sliced, for garnish

Fresh blueberries, for garnish

* If you accidentally get sweetened soy milk, just reduce the sugar to balance it out. As everyone and their mother says in Southern California, "No worries."

1. Combine water, sugar, soy milk, and almond extract in a pot and bring to a simmer over medium heat while stirring to dissolve the sugar. Once sugar is dissolved and the liquid is warm to the touch, add agar-agar and whisk for 1 minute until it completely dissolves.

2. Pour liquid into a container deep enough for it to set. A rectangular pyrex glass cake pan usually works. Pop the liquid bubbles that will form at the top. Because agar-agar can be notoriously difficult to manage, is "cranky," and won't set correctly if disturbed, do not shake, bump, or move.

3. Let set for 10–15 minutes. Here's the frustrating part: If it doesn't set, you might have to start all over again with a new set of ingredients. (You can try reheating and stirring the mixture over medium-low heat just in case it didn't dissolve correctly. Once it steams, remove from heat and pour back into your mold of choice. If it still doesn't set, reheat and add a touch more agar-agar, and if *that* doesn't work, sorry to say, you have to start over.)

4. After it sets, refrigerate.

When ready to serve, cut into cubes. Serve in a bowl with a generous amount of evaporated milk, strawberries, and blueberries and become One with your inner Chinese child through this classic dessert.

FIVE-SPICE APPLE FRITTERS (FORMERLY KNOWN AS FLUFFY THE APPLE FRITTER AND ITS BANANA JAM SIDEKICK)

I don't think I've ever had an apple fritter that packed the crunch of an apple, in any form, donut or otherwise. I always wondered whether the "apple" was really an apple mix masquerading as the real thing. This is our solution.

BALLS OUT
40–80 SERVINGS

2½ cups plus 1¼ cups sugar

2½ teaspoons five-spice powder

7½ cups flour

7½ cups cornstarch

1⅔ tablespoons Alsa brand baking powder *

10 Granny Smith apples, small dice †

5 (12-ounce) cans Coco Rico brand soda

⅓ teaspoon kosher salt

2–4 SERVINGS

½ cup plus ¼ cup sugar

½ teaspoon five-spice powder

1½ cups flour

1½ cups cornstarch

1 teaspoon Alsa brand baking powder *

2 Granny Smith apples, small dice †

1 (12-ounce) can Coco Rico brand soda

1 pinch kosher salt

Honey Bourbon Cream Sauce (page 243), for garnish and on the side

* This is a special French baking powder. We've never made this recipe using anything else, so if you don't got it, try some other baking powder at your own risk . . . and then tweet us about how it worked.

† Not Fujis, not Galas, not Washingtons—we're looking for that tart kinda apple to complement all the other sweetness this dish already has.

1. Over medium-high heat, heat 2 inches of oil in a pot to 350°F.
2. Combine ½ cup sugar and five-spice powder in a bowl and mix evenly. Set aside. In another bowl, sift together flour, cornstarch, and baking powder. Add to that bowl diced Granny Smith apples, soda, salt, and remaining sugar.
3. Allow all the ingredients to slowly marry each other. After 10–20 minutes, incorporate ever so slightly with a spatula, but don't over mix! Ya gotta make sure those pesky glutens don't get activated by unbelievably abundant "air" such that they stand in the way of the pleasure that "fluffy" will give you (which is what will happen if it's overly mixed and becomes too dense).
4. Once the oil is hot, scoop up batter with an ice cream scoop, then gently drop into oil. Turn the fritters frequently and fry until they turn a nice, mouthwatering golden color. To make sure the fritters are cooked through, stick them with a skewer or toothpick. When

you remove it, it should be completely dry. If it's not, continue to fry. Once the fritters are done, remove and shake off excess oil. Let fritters cool for 2 minutes.

5. Transfer slightly cooled fritters to five-spice sugar mix. Toss gently to coat.

6. Plate and serve with a huge side of Honey Bourbon Cream Sauce. (FYI that stuff is like thick and viscous liquid crack, so give yourself an ample side to smother the fritters and yourself in. You're welcome.)

You can store any unused fritter batter covered in the fridge to fry again another day.

The entire appeal of Starry Kitchen,
other than the food, of course,
was the fact that it was hard to find,
that it was underground.

—THE RESTAURANT IN APARTMENT NO. 205

〰〰

BLACK SESAME PANNA COTTA

I love all our panna cottas as if they were my children . . . but this COULD be my fave, even if I said something else somewhere, because . . . GREEN TEA LEMON LATTE COOKIES! (I'm a sucker for cookies.)

BALLS OUT

40–80 SERVINGS

9 tablespoons gelatin powder or 27 bronze gelatin sheets/leaves

3 cups plus 6 cups heavy whipping cream

9 cups whole milk

1⅔ cups black sesame powder

3⅓ cups sugar

Green Tea Lemon Latte Cookies (page 153)

2–4 SERVINGS

1 tablespoon gelatin powder or 3 bronze gelatin sheets/leaves

½ cup plus 1 cup heavy whipping cream

1½ cups whole milk

3 tablespoons black sesame powder

6 tablespoons sugar

Green Tea Lemon Latte Cookies (page 153)

1. If using gelatin sheets, add to a bowl of ice-cold water and submerge. Soak (aka let the gelatin bloom) for 5–7 minutes, or until they soften. To prevent sheets from breaking down, drain water immediately after the 5–7 minutes and gently wring out remaining water from the sheets, just like you would wring out a towel.
2. If using powdered gelatin, place gelatin in a bowl and add ½ cup heavy cream. Let sit and bloom.
3. If using a mold to shape and pop out your panna cotta, brush a light layer of cooking oil on the bottom and sides.
4. This next step is very delicate because gelatin in any form is fairly unstable, so this may take some trial and error, based on a balance of your heat and your feel for that heat. You'll know what I mean if you mess up. If you don't, you're a natural-born talent!
5. Heat sugar, milk, and remaining heavy cream in a pot on medium-low heat until sugar dissolves and liquid is warm to the touch. It should be close to steaming, but definitely not boiling. If you have a thermometer, DO NOT go over 145°F. Next, add gelatin (sheets or powdered heavy cream) and whisk until gelatin dissolves. Add black sesame powder and continue to whisk. This will take a few minutes.
6. Once the sesame powder is incorporated, remove from heat and strain through a chinois or fine mesh strainer to get a silky consistency.

7. Fill your molds, ramekins, or whatever way you want to eat 'em. In between pours, mix pot well to prevent the panna cotta from settling and black sesame from separating. This panna cotta version settles very quickly.

8. To get the most silky consistency possible for each panna cotta, let the molds sit at room temperature for 30–45 minutes. A thin film—a super-high butterfat concentration of milk, cream, black sesame, and gelatin—will form on the surface. Remove the film by gliding a small fork gently over the surface. Collect film in a small bowl and refrigerate overnight along with the panna cotta. Serve panna cotta with Green Tea Lemon Latte Cookies.

To best enjoy that deliciously rich film, mix it into a consistent paste and spread it on bread, toast, or other savories—TWO desserts for the price of one!

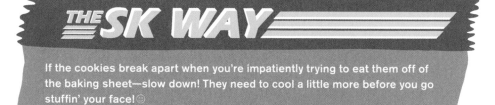

THE SK WAY

If the cookies break apart when you're impatiently trying to eat them off of the baking sheet—slow down! They need to cool a little more before you go stuffin' your face!☺

GREEN TEA LEMON LATTE COOKIES

Delicious! ☺

BALLS OUT
40–80 SERVINGS

9 cups flour

1 tablespoon baking powder*

3 pinches kosher salt

3 tablespoons green tea latte powder†

3 tablespoons lemon zest

3 cups (1½ pounds) unsalted butter, softened to room temperature

3 cups sugar

3 large eggs, room temperature

Powdered sugar, for rolling dough

2–4 SERVINGS

3 cups flour

1 teaspoon baking powder*

Pinch of kosher salt

1 tablespoon green tea latte powder†

1 tablespoon lemon zest

1 cup (½ pound) unsalted butter, softened to room temperature

1 cup sugar

1 large egg, room temperature

Powdered sugar, for rolling dough

* Don't mix this up with baking soda, sucka. That's COMPLETELY different.

† Not tea leaves, more like matcha/green tea powder. We like to use an instant green tea latte powder mix, because it tastes GOOOOOOOOD.

1. Preheat oven to 350°F.
2. Combine flour, baking powder, salt, green tea latte powder, and lemon zest in a bowl. Whisk together then set aside.
3. When butter is room temperature, combine with sugar in a bowl and mix—either with a stand mixer (paddle attachment), with a hand mixer, or with a spatula or wooden spoon. If it's not blending together easily and is lumpy, your butter just ain't soft enough! Patience with butter is key here—and key to becoming a better *Street Fighter II* player too (I'm pretty decent now). Better dough. Better spread. (FYI—best time to stick yer finger in and "taste test" . . . just because.)
4. Add egg and mix together. Next, slowly fold in flour; (may I re-emphasize) FOLD until fully incorporated. The dough will form quickly. When it forms a ball and starts to pull away from the bowl easily, that dough is read-ay!
5. Generously coat a clean surface with powdered sugar for rolling out the dough. Smooth out dough on that surface with a rolling pin.

The dough should be ¼ inch thick. Use a cute cookie cutter of your choice (I'm going to choose . . . TOTORO, so cute!), and cut out as many cookies as you can from the dough. You're honestly free to cut them in any size, but if you're making this to go with Black Sesame Panna Cotta, the daintier the better.

6. Reconstitute and combine uncut dough by hand, roll out to ¼ inch thick, and cut more cookies. (FYI—the reconstituted dough cookies will get more dense the more you do this, but wasting good cookie dough is an international crime . . . or at least should be.)

Place cookies on a baking sheet with parchment paper, a Silpat, or some butter with a light coat of flour, about 1½ inches apart. Bake in preheated oven on middle rack for 8–10 minutes or until golden (and not doughy looking). Remove, let cool. Serve.

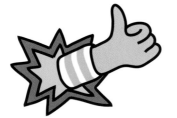

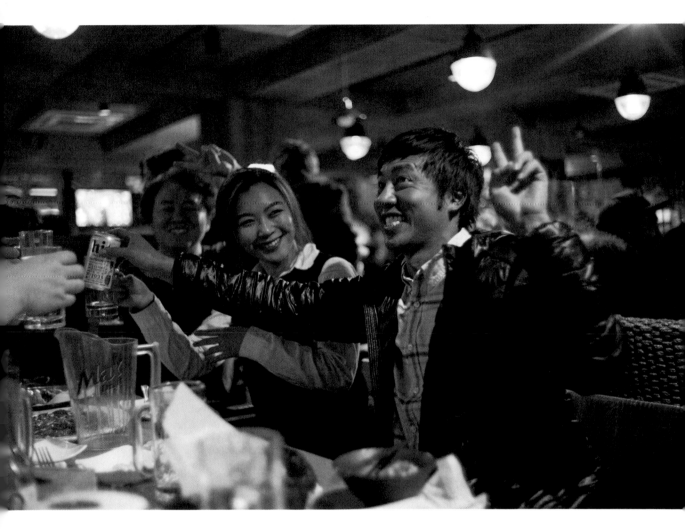

THE *THAI PROSTITUTE* WHO INTRODUCED ME TO PANDAN/KAYA

A LOT OF CREEPY OLD WHITE GUYS GO TO THAILAND TO FIND YOUNG FEMALE COMPANIONS. I'M NOT GOING TO JUDGE ANYONE FOR THEIR QUESTIONABLE MORAL BEHAVIOR, OR GET INTO THE POLITICS OF THE INTERNATIONAL SEX TRADE, BUT I CAN ABSOLUTELY TELL YOU THAT MY THREE—AND ONLY THREE—FAVORITE THINGS ABOUT THAILAND ARE AS FOLLOWS, WRITTEN OUT FOR YOU IN A HANDY TRAVEL-WEBSITE-STYLE LISTICLE:

1. Thailand is literally the cheapest international vacation you can take. I mean, you can see a lot, eat a lot, and not really break the bank . . . Seriously, it's cheap.

2. People are so nice and honest here. No sarcasm. No joke. Thai folks are about the nicest people you will ever hope to meet. I remember mistakenly thinking someone had stolen my camera. Instead of ignoring my plea for help, they helped me find my camera!

3. Thailand is home to one of my all-of-my-lifetime (and should-be-yours) favorite desserts. And I just happened to have discovered it with the help of a prostitute. Let me explain.

At the end of 2005, my future in-laws persuaded me and Thi to join them on a trip to Hong Kong to visit family. We also planned to go to Thailand on their recommendation, where they Asian-parent-insisted (which is more of a command than a recommendation) we join a tour, which I DEPLORE AND STAND VEHEMENTLY AGAINST when I travel. But tours in Thailand are unlike tours anywhere else in the world. That's partly because being a tour guide in Thailand requires a full-fledged degree one earns at school. And we're not talking about a six-week course. We're talking a full-time, four-year program, like a bachelor's degree here in the States. Tourism is the BIGGEST business in Thailand, which also makes the Tourism Authority of Thailand (TAT) one of the—if not *the*—most powerful governmental bodies in the country. Even if you loathe tours like me, you have to take tours in Thailand seriously; they're definitely worth your consideration.

About a month and a half later, a film I was working on called *Journey from the Fall* was selected for the Bangkok Film Festival. I was excited to return to Thailand, now that I was a veteran of the Thai experience—you know, because of all of the five days I had spent there LOL. We stayed in an area right next to Siam Paragon, a famous shopping center that attracts a lot of expats. Though I didn't notice it much at first, the overwhelming presence of tourists in our district tipped us off to the fact that there was a club in the basement of our hotel. And that club had literally one guy for every twenty to thirty girls, who I realized were prostitutes—ex-pat town!

One night, after eating, drinking, and karaoke-ing our hearts out at the film festival, my curiosity got the best of me and I ventured into this unknown clubland filled a-plenty with hookers galore—oh boy!

I should mention here that my previous trip to Asia had changed the way I viewed myself. Up until that point, I had always been insecure about my looks, basically because I'm not a tall, chiseled white guy. I'm kinda sorta gaysianly (oh, it's a thing if you don't know already) youthful looking, and I didn't know this was a thing any woman was into because Asian males are frankly emasculated in the Western world. (I could write a whole book about my insecurities on that topic, but I won't because Asian males are the hot ticket these

days, kid—*high-five*.) But when I had walked around Asia two months before, I had been propositioned, cat-called, and hit on everywhere I went, usually right in front of Thi.

This was at the front of my mind as I entered this club. Which meant that I walked into it with the clear intention of FUCKING with these prostitutes. I don't mean in the sexy-time sense, but in the sense that I knew they thought they were the predators and I was their unsuspecting prey . . . but no, I was the game master and they were my pawns in a game I made up, "fishing for hookers" (I know, I'm twisted). It was pretty simple: I would walk in, looking all innocent, let these women chat me up, and when they tried to proposition me, I'd just coyly laugh and walk away. Now in hindsight, this was pretty cruel, something that I realized by the end of the night, given everything that transpired. But at that moment, with nothing else going on, I was having a great time.

For some reason, one young and seemingly more-impressionable-than-I-looked prostitute piqued my curiosity. She and I started talking, and when she propositioned me, instead of walking away, I shook my head, rubbed my tummy with my left hand, and used my right to mimic eating, and told her I was "hungry!" So I made *her* a proposition. If she didn't go home with any guy that night, I'd buy her dinner, on one condition: She had to take me to her favorite late-night spot, one I never could have found on my own. Like most professionals hoping to separate you from your money, she agreed.

That club wasn't huge, but it was so packed full of women that if you didn't scoop up the one you liked right then and there, you would probably never find her ever again. Nonetheless, about forty-five minutes later, I miraculously found the girl I had propositioned in the ocean of perfume, pushed-up boobs, short skirts, and enough latex hidden in those little purses to cover a football field. She propositioned me one more time, and I reiterated that I was "hungry." We left the club and jumped into a tuk-tuk.

Now, if I could even remember where in Bangkok we ended up, I still wouldn't tell you. This was one of those experiences that is never meant to be replicated or revisited ever again. The driver dropped us off at a random street stall in the middle of a quiet and deserted Bangkok neighborhood in the shadow of the city's beautiful skyline. I told the girl to order whatever she wanted, that it was my treat. Though she didn't speak much English, and I didn't speak a lick of Thai, after much awkwardness I figured out that she was from a small town about an hour outside of Bangkok outside of Bangkok and that she had a South Korean boyfriend who traveled back and forth from Seoul to visit her. The most heartbreaking and human part of this conversation was that neither her mom nor her boyfriend knew she was a prostitute. She didn't know how or when she would ever tell them. She knew it would break her mother's heart, and she had no idea how her boyfriend would react. YEAH, I literally gathered ALL that without being able to speak her language. This was not what I was expecting.

I also wasn't expecting what came out of the kitchen shortly after our heart-to-heart. My horrible phonetic-ization of the Thai would be *ka-ram-pang-song-ka-ya.* The end of that is the part that many Westerners might recognize—*kaya,* or

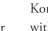

kaya toast, or in this case, kaya bread. It's a mix of egg yolk, coconut cream, and *pandan,* a long green leaf in Southeast Asia that's like vanilla but a little nuttier, used in sweet and savory dishes alike for its incredible aroma and because it changes everything to a super pretty bright green color. And all of that is married to create a thick custardy delicious spread in a bowl served with triangular pieces of white bread. It's kind of a sweet dish, kind of an appetizer, and all you do is take the super-moist bread and dip it into and drench it in the kaya and stuff that deliciousness into your mouth.

HO . . . LY . . . FUCK! It was SO GOOD . . . SO TASTY. So satisfying after a night out. It's so simple, and so comfortingly delicious. And I'm sure that being under the stars in Bangkok with my non-sexual partner in crime for the night didn't hurt either.

This surreal night was incredibly influential in my life because I discovered one of my favorite things in the world (so much so that I sought it out in Thai Town in LA *immediately* after I got back).

I have that young woman to thank—for sharing with me, an arrogant stranger. She gave me more perspective on the world in a short conversation than I ever expected and sent me away with inspiration.

After we finished eating, I put her in a tuk-tuk and sent her home. I looked up at the sky, took everything in, and then went back to the hotel, thinking about that young woman, hoping she would someday marry her South Korean boyfriend and make her mom proud with lots and lots of grandchildren.

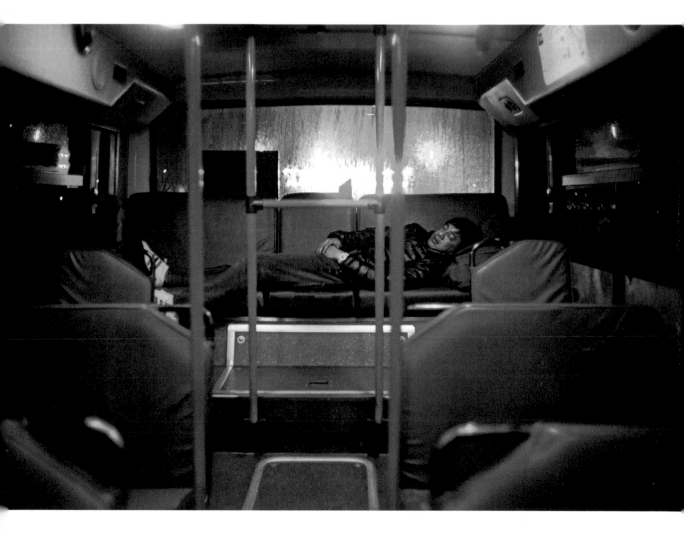

PANDAN CHURROS

These Pandan Churros are the bane of our existence but also one of our most beloved desserts, winning lots of recognition and even a few awards. We probably tried at least thirty different recipes for this lil green dessert—eggless, milkless, and everything in between—to discover something we liked.

BALLS OUT
40–80 SERVINGS

2⅓ cups plus
2 tablespoons unsalted
butter or oil

3⅓ teaspoons vanilla
extract

2½ teaspoons pandan
extract

1⅔ tablespoons
kosher salt

6⅔ tablespoons sugar

10 cups all-purpose flour

10 cups whole milk

40 large eggs

2–4 SERVINGS

2 tablespoons unsalted
butter or oil

½ teaspoon vanilla
extract

⅛ teaspoon pandan
extract

¼ teaspoon kosher salt

1 teaspoon sugar

½ cup all-purpose flour

½ cup whole milk

2 large eggs

Powdered sugar

Coconut Kaya Cream
(page 162), on the side

1. Combine butter, vanilla, pandan, salt, and sugar in a pan over medium-low heat. Dissolve sugar and salt thoroughly in the pan. Once it's all one tasty homogenous mix, steadily fold in flour with a wooden or high-temperature-rated spatula until dough congeals into one big ball.

2. Remove from heat and let cool for 10–15 minutes. Before proceeding to the next step, double- and triple-check to make sure the dough isn't warm at all.

3. Heat 2 inches of oil in a pot over medium-high heat to 350°F.

4. While waiting for the oil to heat, add eggs to the dough, one egg at a time, folding in each egg until fully incorporated.

5. Now we have some options for how we form and fry the churro.

   - If you happen to have a cranking churrera churro maker OR a similar sausage machine (no joke, some are one and the same), use that with the hollow attachment and crank away!

   - If you're a baker and have a piping bag for icing and such, use that with a star tip and pipe away!

   - If you don't have either of those but you do have a plastic resealable freezer bag, with a pair of scissors cut a hole 1 inch in diameter diagonally across one of the bottom corners of the bag.

This will be your piping bag. It won't work as well unless it's a *freezer* bag because they tend to be thicker and stronger. Word of advice: The bag still won't last long because as you start applying pressure, the bag will eventually tear. So have a couple of bags handy.

6. Finally, if you don't have any of *that* stuff or the inclination to find out whether you do, you'll have to go without fancy shapes—but you can roll your own long cylindrical tubes.

7. Once the oil is hot, drop your churros in the oil and fry for 2 minutes per side. Be sure to turn over often to check the color. When finished, churros will come out a beautiful green and brownish color. Try one out. It should be fluffy and tasty.

    Plate it, sprinkle on powdered sugar, and serve with a side of extra creamy and custardy Coconut Kaya Cream.

Against ALL odds and especially when I'm fucked, I get shit done. I don't cave in.

—CHAOS AND PORK CHOP SANDWICHES

〰

COCONUT KAYA CREAM

This is the delicious other half of kaya toast, the CREEEEEEEEEEEAMY part. Kaya is usually pandan, coconut, and eggs, so if you want to get fancy, when you combine it with our Pandan Churros, it's basically kaya . . . DECONSTRUCTED. Did that sound Top Chef-y enough?

BALLS OUT
40–80 SERVINGS

7½ cups coconut cream

1¾ cups brown sugar

50 large egg yolks

1¾ cups sugar

2–4 SERVINGS

¾ cup coconut cream	5 large egg yolks	8½ teaspoons sugar
8½ teaspoons brown sugar		

1. Combine coconut cream and brown sugar in a small pot. Heat over low heat until brown sugar dissolves. Remove from heat and set aside.
2. In a separate bowl, whisk together egg yolks and sugar. Gradually whisk in melted brown sugar and coconut cream until the two become . . . one!
3. Return pot to low heat and stir with a rubber spatula or spoon for 5–10 minutes, or until custard thickens and you can dip a spoon in, pull it out, and draw your finger cleanly across the back of the spoon. That's technique, SON! Just a reminder—DO NOT BOIL.
4. Remove from heat, strain sauce through a chinois or fine mesh strainer, constantly running liquid through and around the chinois with the spatula. It should be a beautiful yellow color.

   Let it cool. Cover and refrigerate. Dip every pastry in it and enjoy.

THE SK WAY

Save your egg whites to make Sweet and Sour Ribeye Beef (page 162) or Triple-Cooked Osmanthus Pork Spareribs (page 170). Store them in the fridge up to 2 to 4 days.

SWEET AND SOUR RIBEYE BEEF

I like to call this dish, "Not yo' momma's Chinese take-out." Contrary to belief, this very popular dish IS in fact an actual Chinese dish made with a homemade sauce. For those of you who knew that or didn't doubt it, good on you! For those of you who still don't believe it, BELIEVE!

2–4 SERVINGS

6 ounces ribeye beef, cut into thin 2-inch-long strips

½ head(s) of frisee or purple kale, cleaned and root trimmed

SAUCE:

1 cup sugar

6 tablespoons light soy sauce

1 cup plus 2 tablespoons water

½ cup rice vinegar

2 tablespoons roasted sesame oil

2 tablespoons crushed red pepper flakes

½ cup minced ginger

3⅓ tablespoons minced garlic

¼ tablespoon chopped scallions

¼ tablespoon shredded carrots

2 tablespoons tapioca starch

BATTER:

1 large egg white

1 pinch kosher salt

1 pinch black pepper

1 pinch mushroom bouillon

½ cup cornstarch

BALLS OUT
40–80 SERVINGS

7½ pounds ribeye beef, cut into thin 2-inch-long strips

10 heads of frisee or purple kale, cleaned and root trimmed

SAUCE:

3 cups sugar

1 cups plus 2 tablespoons light soy sauce

3 cups plus 6 tablespoons water

1½ cups rice vinegar

6 tablespoons roasted sesame oil

⅓ cup crushed red pepper flakes

1½ cups minced ginger

⅔ cup minced garlic

¾ tablespoon chopped scallions

¾ tablespoon shredded carrots

6 tablespoons tapioca starch

BATTER:

10 egg whites

1¼ teaspoons mushroom bouillon

1¼ teaspoons black pepper

1¼ teaspoons kosher salt

5 cups cornstarch

1. First, a note: Please love your ribeye and do not cut in the same direction as the beef striations/lines. Cut directly across/perpendicular to/90 degrees from the lines. This is the single most important note for assuring that you get the most tender strips possible. Also, make sure all your strips are fairly uniform so you'll have a fairly uniform cook time, too. If you don't, you'll have a wide range of uncooked beef and overcooked beef, which will become a crazy circus of confusingly different textures in your mouth!

2. Dissolve sugar in soy sauce and 1 cup water over low heat. Once completely dissolved, mix in rice vinegar, sesame oil, and red pepper flakes. Keep sauce warm over low heat. In a separate pan, sauté ginger and garlic together with a little bit of cooking oil over medium-high heat, then add to sauce. Next, sauté scallions and carrots with cooking oil over medium-high heat. Stir into sauce.

3. Next, make your thickening slurry for the sauce by mixing your remaining water and tapioca in a small bowl. Make sure it's very well mixed and incorporated. Lightly thicken the sauce by slowly adding a little bit of tapioca slurry at a time (don't use all of it if you can help it) and mixing in often until you get a medium-thick consistency to coat the battered beef with later on. Hold the sauce over lowest heat.

4. Place the egg white into a small bowl. Combine salt, pepper, mushroom bouillon, and cornstarch in another bowl and mix together.

5. Dip beef strips into egg white wash, shake off excess, and then aggressively coat in the batter bowl of cornstarch mix.

6. Heat 1 inch cooking oil in a pot to 350°F. When the oil is ready, gently place your battered beef strips in the oil. For the first 10 seconds, let them strips fry free. After that, start stirring and breaking apart the beef to make sure the strips don't stick together ("stay away!"). Cook for a total of 35–45 seconds. Remove beef, drain, and shake off excess oil over pot for about 15 seconds and then fry once more for another 20–30 seconds, or until beef is crispy. Remove, shake off the oil one more time, and transfer to a bowl.

   Remove thickened sauce pot from heat, transfer ½ cup sauce to a separate bowl, and store the rest—cool off, cover, and refrigerate to be used another time. Toss crispy beef strips in sauce bowl and lightly coat the beef. Remove and plate on a bed of fancy-ass frisee or your favorite leafy vegetable, and go . . . to . . . TOWN!

HANOI GRILLED TURMERIC FISH WITH DILL AND ONION

This is quite literally the "other" favorite dish I discovered as a Vietnamese adult (the first being the *Bun Cha Hanoi* aka Hanoi Grilled Pork Belly and Pork Patty). Our version is a little variation on the OG dish, which I devoured in Hanoi for the book and . . . holy CRAP was it GOOD! So, feel free to experiment and try out other variations.

BALLS OUT
40–80 SERVINGS

3⅔ cups fish sauce

6⅔ tablespoons turmeric powder

1¼ cups minced garlic

10 tablespoons fresh ginger

2½ cups finely diced shallots

1¼ cups chopped dill fronds

5 teaspoons ground black pepper

20 pounds striped bass skin-on fish filets, or any kind of white fish

20 small yellow or white onions, diced

6⅔ bunch plus 13⅓ bunch fresh dill, stemmed

40 plus 40 scallion stalks, cut into 2-inch pieces

10 cups roasted peanuts, coarsely chopped

10 pounds (160 ounces) vermicelli, cooked

2–4 SERVINGS

3 tablespoons fish sauce

1 teaspoon turmeric powder

1 tablespoon minced garlic

½ tablespoon fresh ginger

2 tablespoons finely diced shallots

1 tablespoon chopped dill fronds

¼ teaspoon ground black pepper

1 pound striped bass skin-on fish filets, or any kind of white fish

1 small yellow or white onion, sliced

⅓ bunch plus ⅔ bunch fresh dill, stemmed

2 plus 2 scallion stalks, cut into 2-inch pieces

Persian cucumber, julienned

Pickled Red Onions (page 249)

½ cup roasted peanuts, coarsely chopped

8 ounces vermicelli, cooked

Coco Rico Vietnamese Fish Sauce (page 240)

Butter lettuce

"Mam Nem" (optional)

---

1. Mix fish sauce, turmeric powder, garlic, ginger, shallots, dill fronds, and black pepper in a bowl. Add fish and coat evenly. Cover and refrigerate for no longer than 30 minutes, or else the fish will get too salty as you prepare the rest of the recipe.

2. Heat a little bit of oil on high heat in a pan/skillet and sauté onions until lightly golden. Add ⅓ bunch of fresh dill and two sliced scallions stalks to the party. Sauté for an additional 1–2 minutes. Plate the onions, scallions, and dill on a serving platter.

3. Remove fish from bowl, drain, and dispose of marinade. Pat dry excess marinade with paper towels so the sugar in the fish sauce doesn't burn the fish.

4. In the same pan used to cook the onions, heat a little more oil on medium-high heat. Pan-fry the fish for 3–4 minutes, or until both

sides are evenly browned. If you have delicious skin-on fish, give some extra cooking love to that skin, which should turn nice and crispy before you flip it.

5. Plate the fish on sautéed onions, scallions, and dill. Garnish with remaining fresh dill and scallions, cucumber, Pickled Red Onions, and peanuts.

Serve immediately with sides of vermicelli noodles, Coco Rico Vietnamese Fish Sauce, and butter lettuce. Wrap everything, eat everything in a bowl, or whatever combination makes you happy. (I and many Vietnamese especially like it with "Mam Nem", a fermented fish and pineapple dipping sauce—don't knock it til you try it!) Enjoy one of my favoritest dishes evaaaaaaaaaaaaaaaaaaaar!

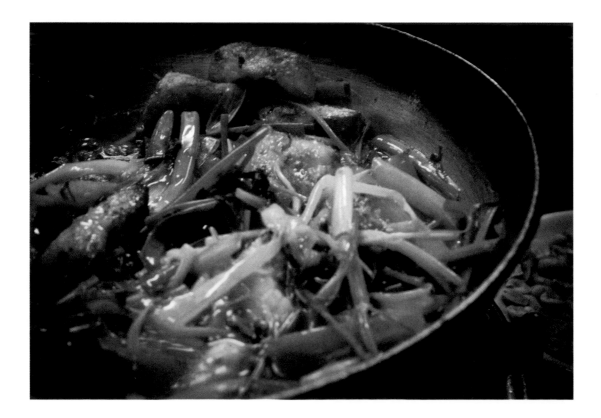

BUN CHA HANOI (AKA HANOI GRILLED PORK BELLY AND PORK PATTY)

A former special and now a staple dish of our menu, this is one of my two favorite dishes that I discovered as a Vietnamese adult—way before Anthony Bourdain and President Barack Obama made this even MORE famous. Traditionally, this is a noodle dish (hence the Vietnamese word for vermicelli, *bun*, in the name), where you grab a portion of noodles for yourself in a small bowl, add hand-torn herbs and lettuce and whatever pork you like, and drizzle the fish sauce the pork is swimming in all over your noodles.

BALLS OUT
40–80 SERVINGS

10 pounds pork belly, sliced

10 pounds ground pork

10 tablespoons minced garlic

10 tablespoons oyster sauce

10 tablespoons sugar

1 cup plus 4 tablespoons fish sauce

1 cup plus 4 tablespoons minced shallots

1 cup plus 4 tablespoons minced lemongrass

1 cup plus 4 tablespoons Caramel Sauce (page 239)

3⅓ tablespoons chicken bouillon

5 teaspoons ground black pepper

DIPPING SAUCE:

2½ cups fish sauce

2½ cups sugar

15 cups water

2–4 SERVINGS

1 pound pork belly, sliced

1 pound ground pork

1 tablespoon minced garlic

1 tablespoon oyster sauce

1 tablespoon sugar

2 tablespoons fish sauce

2 tablespoons minced shallots

2 tablespoons minced lemongrass

2 tablespoons Caramel Sauce (page 239)

1 teaspoon chicken bouillon

½ teaspoon ground black pepper

DIPPING SAUCE:

¼ cup fish sauce

¼ cup sugar

1½ cups water

FINAL PRODUCT AND GARNISHES:

Rice vermicelli noodles

Pickled Watermelon Rinds (page 251)

Mint, cleaned and stemmed

Cilantro, cleaned

Pickled Kohlrabi (page 246)

Butter lettuce*

* No two types of lettuce are the same (except Boston lettuce IS butter lettuce). Use butter lettuce because it gives a great crunch to the dish and holds up well, too. Oh, and you can wrap really well with it if you wanna WRAP!

1. Combine pork belly and ground pork with garlic, oyster sauce, sugar, fish sauce, shallots, lemongrass, Caramel Sauce, chicken bouillon, and pepper in a bowl. Mix, marinate, and refrigerate for 3–4 hours, or overnight if you want maximum flavor penetration.
2. When the pork is ready, form eight 2-inch patties with the ground pork, lay flat on a tray, and set aside.
3. Combine fish sauce, sugar, and water in a pot. Heat under medium-low heat, stirring until sugar dissolves. Fill a serving bowl halfway

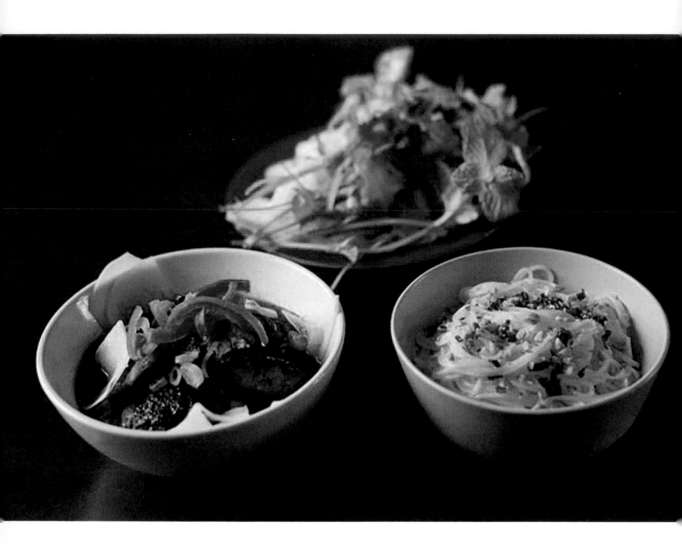

with it. Keep the rest in the pot over low heat, or let it cool off, transfer to a container, cover, and store in the refrigerator.

4. Next, bring water to boil in a large pot over high heat. When water boils, drop in vermicelli and cook for about 1 minute. Rinse under cold water and shake off excess; transfer to a common bowl for everyone to share.

5. If you have a grill, bring up to a medium-high flame and cook patties and pork belly for 3–4 minutes on each side, or until the meat cooks through and has a nice set of grill marks.

   If you don't have a grill, sauté patties and pork belly in a pan/wok with some oil for about 3–5 minutes for each side or until they're cooked through. Transfer patties and pork belly to the half-filled bowl of fish sauce. Top with Pickled Watermelon Rinds to add a lil spice o' color. Complement all this pork-liciousness with vermicelli on butter lettuce and serve with mint, cilantro, and a side of Pickled Kohlrabi, a platter of Vietnamese fixin's. Enjoy the Vietnamese dish that makes me feel like I'm all grown(s) up!

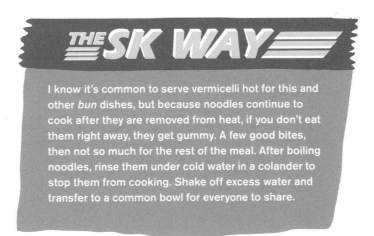

THE SK WAY

I know it's common to serve vermicelli hot for this and other *bun* dishes, but because noodles continue to cook after they are removed from heat, if you don't eat them right away, they get gummy. A few good bites, then not so much for the rest of the meal. After boiling noodles, rinse them under cold water in a colander to stop them from cooking. Shake off excess water and transfer to a common bowl for everyone to share.

TRIPLE-COOKED OSMANTHUS PORK SPARERIBS

I DON'T have a good story about this dish. I don't really have a good way to describe it, even as talky as I am. What *is* good, however, in addition to the dish, is the versatility of osmanthus, which can be used in Osmanthus Panna Cotta and with ribs because it straddles the line between sweet and savory. This dish IS cooked THREE times: Slow-roasted, fried, then spectacularly sautéed in a funky-on-its-own but amazing-when-combined-and-served-with a fresh pineapple sauce.

2–4 SERVINGS

2 tablespoons sugar

2 tablespoons fish sauce

1 tablespoon plus
1 tablespoon minced garlic

¼ cup finely chopped shallots

1 teaspoon kosher salt

1 pound pork spareribs *

1 cup (~8 large eggs) egg whites

1 cup flour

1 cup cornstarch

1 teaspoon mushroom bouillon

1 teaspoon kosher salt

1 teaspoon black pepper

FOR STIR-FRYIN':

1 red bell pepper, medium diced

½ cup 1-inch cubes fresh

pineapple

1 tablespoon rice vinegar

1 tablespoon chicken bouillon

3 tablespoons osmanthus syrup, plus additional for flavor

1 teaspoon kosher salt

OSMANTHUS SYRUP:

½ cup water

⅓ cup sugar

2 tablespoons osmanthus flower

* Baby back ribs, or any kind of pork riblets, work, but spareribs are less prissy, more marbly meaty, and more downright ugly-licious than others.

BALLS OUT
40–80 SERVINGS

2⅓ cups plus
2 tablespoons sugar

2⅓ cups plus
2 tablespoons fish sauce

1 cup plus 4 tablespoons minced garlic

5 cups finely chopped shallots

6⅔ tablespoons kosher salt

20 pounds pork spareribs *

5 quarts (~160 large eggs) egg whites

5 quarts flour

5 quarts cornstarch

6⅔ tablespoons mushroom bouillon

6⅔ tablespoons kosher salt

6⅔ tablespoons black pepper

FOR STIR-FRYIN':

20 red bell peppers, medium diced

10 cups 1-inch cubes fresh pineapple

1 cup plus 4 tablespoons rice vinegar

1 cup plus 4 tablespoons chicken bouillon

3⅔ cups osmanthus syrup,

plus additional for flavor

6⅔ tablespoons kosher salt

OSMANTHUS SYRUP:

10 cups water

6⅔ cups sugar

2⅓ cups plus
2 tablespoons osmanthus flower

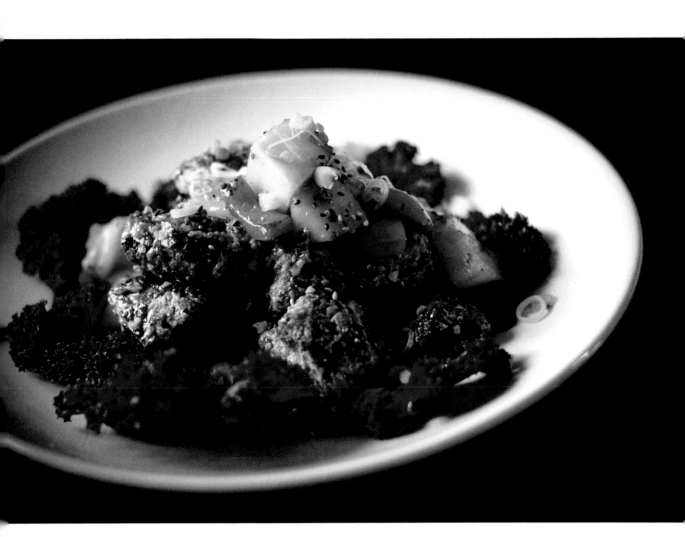

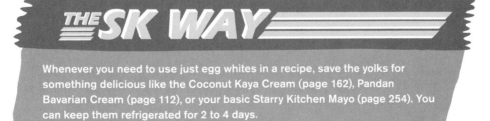

THE SK WAY

Whenever you need to use just egg whites in a recipe, save the yolks for something delicious like the Coconut Kaya Cream (page 162), Pandan Bavarian Cream (page 112), or your basic Starry Kitchen Mayo (page 254). You can keep them refrigerated for 2 to 4 days.

1. **TO MAKE THE OSMANTHUS SYRUP:** Bring water and sugar to boil in a pot over high heat, and mix. When the syrup thickens slightly, reduce to medium heat and add osmanthus flower. Let simmer for 1 minute, then turn off the heat. Let sit and infuse for an additional 5 minutes before using. Strain; remove and dispose of flower.

2. Dissolve sugar in fish sauce in a separate pot over low heat. Once dissolved, add garlic, shallots, and salt. Remove from heat, transfer to a bowl large enough to hold your ribs, and let sauce cool. Once it nears room temperature, add pork ribs, massage in the flavor (and your dreams), and marinate overnight.

3. Preheat oven to 300°F. While waiting for the oven to heat, transfer ribs into a cake pan or something similar that can be safely covered; lay ribs out in a single layer and cover. (Completely wrapping in foil works, if you don't have a proper lid.)

4. Once the oven is ready, place covered ribs on the middle rack for 2½ hours. Check often to make sure the meat's not falling off the bone, because it's more difficult to cook the meat two more times without the bones for support.

5. Remove from oven, drain all those fantastic juices (but really, save those juices for some original fried rice concoction, and then Instagram us), and set aside to cool.

6. Heat 2 inches of oil in a sturdy pot on high heat to 350°F. Next, prepare your egg white "wash" in a bowl. In a separate bowl, mix flour, cornstarch, mushroom bouillon, salt, and pepper. Taste it, adjust seasoning as needed, and get ready to dredge!

7. Once the oil is hot, dip each rib individually in the egg white wash, shake off excess, then dredge thoroughly in the flour mix and all around (Imagine it being like a fancy slow-mo Red Lobster commercial, like I do!).

8. Then drop in oil and . . . FRY AWAY for about 4–5 minutes, or until the outside turns golden and crunchy. Remove, shake off excess oil, and drip dry on a towel or grated baking sheet.

9. Next, sauté bell peppers and pineapple in a pan with a little bit of oil on high heat until slightly browned. Add rice vinegar, chicken bouillon, remaining garlic, osmanthus syrup, and salt. Mix everything into one consistent sauce and stir-fry, then add the ribs. Toss and sauté quickly, fully coating the ribs and sealing in that flavor with the heat of your pan. Make sure ribs are hot, then plate and serve with rice.

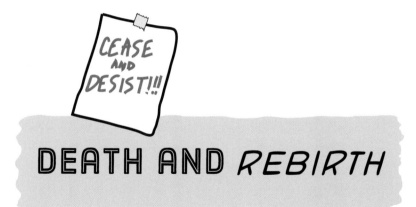

DEATH AND *REBIRTH*

The difference between this email and the millions of other emails I receive about business opportunities was how earnest it was. Reading it, I knew that this fan probably was one of the nicest guys I would ever meet, and I loved how crazy the idea would seem to the outside world—and oh yeah, I own 600+ retro console videogames—so the thought of opening a full restaurant bar arcade really struck a chord in me. Thus the path toward working with Jordan Weiss on Button Mash began—though it took more than three years to come to fruition.

But before that fruition, at the beginning of 2015, we launched a Kickstarter crowd-funding campaign to kick Starry Kitchen into serious overdrive. We decided that if we didn't

reach our goal of $500,000, we would end the restaurant once and for all. Though we raised $115,000, we fell too short.

It was over. We quit. We were burned out. We had accomplished so much, from our apartment in 2009 to leaving on our own terms at the peak of our growth and popularity . . . because we could. A lot of people were perplexed. Why would we stop when we had built a brand that more and more people were discovering? Why would we stop when LA was on the cusp of getting national recognition for what we already knew here at home: LA is the Wild West of food and has an incredible community of personalities and talent that the world hasn't seen before—and we as eaters in LA couldn't give a rat's ass about tablecloths, Michelin stars, or James Beard and his awards! So why did we stop? Because of the simple fact that "happy people make happy food" conversely translates to "unhappy people make . . . ," and we needed to be happy again before we made any more food.

I won't lie. I loved all the time and experiences that came our way during those six years. I didn't love the downs and how it made my Kitchen Ninja wife feel. Those lows got lower and lower each time. After you've experienced the worst day of your life, it takes an incredibly optimistic perspective to believe that every day is going to be better. But what if each day presents itself as even worse than that worst day? That's demoralizing, no matter how optimistic you are. I don't get down often, and those instances that brought us lower and lower still couldn't break me. But watching Thi struggle through them shattered me. In those moments, I understood that I would have to carry the full weight of Starry Kitchen on my own until my beloved Kitchen Ninja could come around. But six years into our exploits, I knew I couldn't play that hand again. Our adventure, at least this version of it, was quickly coming to an end. If we were going to do any more with Starry Kitchen, Thi and I needed to be in step. So we needed to step away. We needed to quit. Maybe for the first time in our relationship, *us* was more important than *me*.

After we stepped away, I did something very unique and contrary to my pushy type-A history. I didn't try to will/persuade/coerce Thi into loving her talent for the food business. I decided I wouldn't even mention the business until she felt like coming 'round—positively or negatively—so I could get her honest not-influenced-by-my-loud-mouth assessment of what she wanted.

'Til then, I did everything I could think of that was free under the sun. I stretched. I hiked. I read. I went to the beach. I caught up with friends. I reflected on the time spent, excited about the time ahead. This was a period of patience—something that has never sat well with me. It took at least a month for my body to understand that it didn't have to fight every day. I was calm. I was willing to take my time pondering the next adventure. And I was willing to wait an eternity to hear what Thi had to say about that next adventure.

During our "funemployment," we started reflecting on the possibility of parenthood. A year earlier we had told our respective parental types that we didn't think kids were in the cards for us; that we had decided not to bring a child into our chaotic lives; that we were content with our life together as we neared our forties. But then three months into our "funemployment," we started trying to have a baby. This change of events also inspired in Thi the revelation that she *did* enjoy making and creating food, that she hadn't been doing it just because I wanted her to.

I'm usually the person who forcefully makes everything into a reality, and it was amazing how time, spiritual room to think, and distance from the responsibility of the restaurant changed everything for us. So we began trying to make a baby after all, and I began thinking about how we could come back onto the food scene.

About one month into baby-making, we came to the weirdly logical realization that

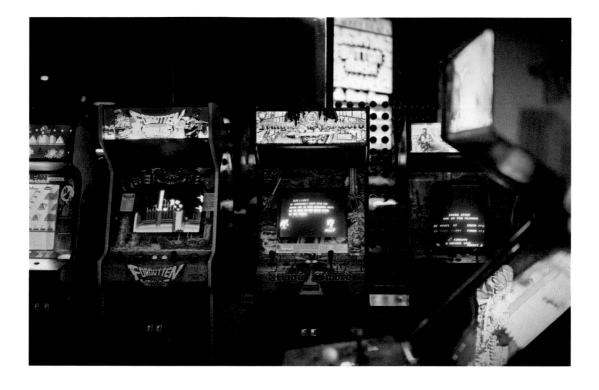

because we were still "funemployed," we didn't have a stable income (or any income, for that matter) and that maybe this wasn't the best time to have a kid just yet. But, as soon as we changed our minds, we found out that Thi Tran was indeed pregnant. This was May 2015. I think Thi was briefly terrified that maybe we weren't ready to have a baby, but I thought it was pretty fucking cool that we had turned on our own decision and logic on its head and . . . we were bringing a little person into this world who would be either the angelic prodigal child or the demon spawn descending on the earth.

So while that pregnancy was going, I came up with an idea that would be Starry Kitchen–esque, completely unexpected, fun, and wide enough to create enough of a stir to

see whether we were in fact still relevant to our beloved LA food scene, or whether we were just an irrelevant relic of the past that needed to put the banana suit and tofu balls to rest and wither and die. That idea: to come back . . . THROUGH UBER!

Short anecdote that makes this far more relevant of an idea that came out of the blue: In Chinatown, through the tutelage of George Yu, the man who held out for two decades to make the new genesis of restaurants in the city happen, I befriended young and talented entrepreneurs, including a new wave of coffee connoisseurs. One was Amnaj, who comes from a well-known Thai family that owns the mega-wholesale store LAX-C, basically the Thai Costco. Amnaj set off on his own to open his own coffee shop, Chimney Coffee. Though I hardly consider myself a coffee historian, I do consider Amnaj part of a uniquely different group of distinguished coffee people who aren't as militant about coffee or so tied to precision as much as they just appreciate great coffee and want to bring as much of it to the masses as they can. One of his ideas was to hold a coffee competition with all the local coffee shops. He invited me to be one of the judges.

At this coffee competition, I met a gentleman by the name of Brian Behrand, who was already a fan of Starry Kitchen's food. And through Brian I met his wife, Eva, head of public affairs at Uber. Brian and Eva were big fans of our Singaporean Chili Crab, and Thi and I randomly ran into them in San Francisco, when we were "funemployed," at Kin Khao, a great Thai restaurant that's right up there with Night+Market and Pok Pok. Seriously.

> I told them from the bottom of my heart, "If Button Mash doesn't work, I'm really quitting this business because I've lost all faith in humanity."
>
> 〰

THIS is what led to the idea that resurrecting Starry Kitchen through Uber could be a reality. Knowing someone on the inside can heighten your confidence and let you believe that any weird idea might become a reality. Which is why I pitched Uber an Uber-unique idea. I developed a full PowerPoint deck with pics, bullet points, and a closing slide of me in my baby blue tux and matching cummerbund. I was giddy, bursting at the seams to frolic in Uberland and scream my idea at the top of the cubicle-less hills there. I packed my banana suit tightly in my backpack and made my way to the LA offices of Uber to make a splash unlike any other seen inside those offices.

But when I arrived at the meeting, they pitched me the exact idea I was about to pitch to them! This wasn't a game we were playing against each other; this was a courtship. I had already won by just walking in. In my many years pitching, peddling, and hustling TV shows, movies, scripts, balls, and all the food we made under the sun, I was used to the uphill battle, the hustle, the battle to persuade the people with the biggest egos to buy into me, my idea, MY BALLS!

It's a rare feeling when someone gets you, let alone reads your thoughts. I was almost in tears.

I got my crew together, and Uber, after much internal debate about my unpredictable exploits (which was understandable☺) finally pulled the trigger and we relaunched via UberEATS in July 2015.

Now the real craziness of this idea was believing we were still relevant enough for people to want our food. To remember who we were. To even care. That was kind of scary. But I did tell Uber to expect me to blow every press relationship I had out of the water. And that I did, along with Uber's huge mailing list of some-odd 50k loyal users in Los Angeles announcing "LA's underground fave Starry Kitchen returns." I got emails, calls, tweets about our surprise announcement. Uber fielded calls about our return every day. They had never seen anything like this. The anticipation was crazy, unpredictable, and . . . it was anyone's guess whether this would actually translate to actual sales of our food.

On July 9th, within the first five minutes of our resurrection John Liu, an executive with UberEATS, told me, "90 percent of your first wave of food is already gone." (There were only two waves of food.) Uber-great for Starry Kitchen, but Uber-bad for UberEATS. I was getting tweets, texts, emails about people who couldn't get through. One of my friends tried for three hours with NO luck. I was laughing and so fucking surprised.

On top of it all, I asked the folks at Uber whether I could deliver in my banana suit—and they said Yes! It was so much fun. At the end of the day, all of it was out of my control . . . because we broke Uber! We broke Uber again the next week EX-CEPT this time we were pissing people off because they couldn't order food no matter how long they waited.

Fortunately, just as UberEATS was becoming less of an experiment and more of an operational reality, Button Mash—the bar arcade that served Asian food (remember where we started?)—was finally picking up steam. With a space secured, a dining room designed, kitchen equipment laid out, all we had to do was wait . . . and wait . . . and wait some more . . . and wait a little longer . . . and even longer . . . and get some lunch . . . and keep waiting for the state to approve our beer + wine license.

So I understand if you have a hard time keeping up with Starry Kitchen's confusing timeline, especially up to this point in our history. Rewinding back to the Kickstarter campaign, our intention was always, "Go big, or go home!" It's important to understand

that Button Mash, though we were definitely involved, was not solely a Starry Kitchen endeavor. Even then, we didn't know how to frame what we were doing for the press and for people because for some reason, creative collab-orations for the public seem finite, a one-off, maybe even a stunt.

The Kickstarter campaign was the time to get everyone out of the dark, take the tough love, tough opinions, tough everything because if there's another shitty rule I try to convey, it's that nothing good in life comes easy, and going on the path to almost-closing had to be an

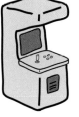

honest exercise for our fans and every-one behind the scenes alike.

Button Mash accidentally became the second stage of Starry Kitchen's resurrection. And it couldn't have come at a better time or arrived with a bigger splash—in branding, spirit, staff, and culture. Without any real press, any real word of mouth, on our first night—a Wednesday—five hundred people came through our doors. Then six hundred the next night. And seven hundred the next. On Satur-day night, we served close to a thousand, which was un-fucking-believable, because as anyone who's ever opened a new business knows, NO ONE KNOWS whether anyone is going to come through those doors.

While I trained my staff, I told them from the bottom of my heart, "If Button Mash doesn't work, I'm really quitting this business because I've lost all faith in humanity." After our opening weekend, Ashley, one of my serv-ers, greeted me with a big smile and hug and said, "Well, I guess you don't have to quit the business."

SPICY KOREAN NOODLES

Our close friend Matt Kim, who gets us all the fresh uni we want (Yay!) introduced us to the original Korean noodle dish—*jjol myeon*. That dish uses a super chewy noodle, but we found these awesomely fresh and chewy ramen noodles by the famous Sun Noodle company, which makes ramen noodles for almost every ramen shop in all of the United States . . . and now for us and these amazingly vegan (without the egg at least) noodles!

2–4 SERVINGS

THE SAUCE:

6 tablespoons *gochujang* (remember, no two cheap *gochujangs* are the same)

2 tablespoons light soy sauce

6 tablespoons rice vinegar

3 tablespoons sesame oil*

4 tablespoons honey

2 tablespoons brown sugar

2 teaspoons Korean chili pepper powder

2 tablespoons toasted white sesame seeds

1 tablespoon Chinese sesame paste

NOODLES AND ALL:

8 ounces fresh ramen noodles or 11 ounces dry noodles (refer to Garlic Noodle recipe, page 25, for notes, options, and thoughts on other noodles)

¼ cup sauce

¼ Asian pear, julienned

¼ Persian cucumber, julienned

3 scallions, julienned

3 thin watermelon slices cut into triangles†

Pickled Watermelon Rinds (page 251)

Toasted white sesame seeds, for garnish

1 soft-boiled egg (optional)

* But really, Japanese or Korean roasted sesame oil is pretty spectacular for this dish.

† Use any leftover watermelon, if there is any, to make some Pickled Watermelon Rinds and/or Watermelon Ginger Agua Fresca and have yerself a watermelon hoedown. *hi-5*

BALLS OUT
40–80 SERVINGS

THE SAUCE:

3⅔ cups *gochujang*

2⅓ cups plus 2 tablespoons light soy sauce

3⅔ cups rice vinegar

1¾ cups plus 1 tablespoon sesame oil*

2⅓ cups plus 2 tablespoons honey

2⅓ cups plus 2 tablespoons brown sugar

6⅔ tablespoons Korean chili pepper powder

2⅓ cups plus 2 tablespoons toasted white sesame seeds

½ cup plus 2 tablespoons Chinese sesame paste

NOODLES AND ALL:

10 pounds fresh ramen noodles or 13¾ pounds dry noodles

5 cups sauce

5 Asian pear, julienned

5 Persian cucumbers, julienned

60 scallions, julienned

20 thin triangles watermelon†

20 soft-boiled eggs (optional)

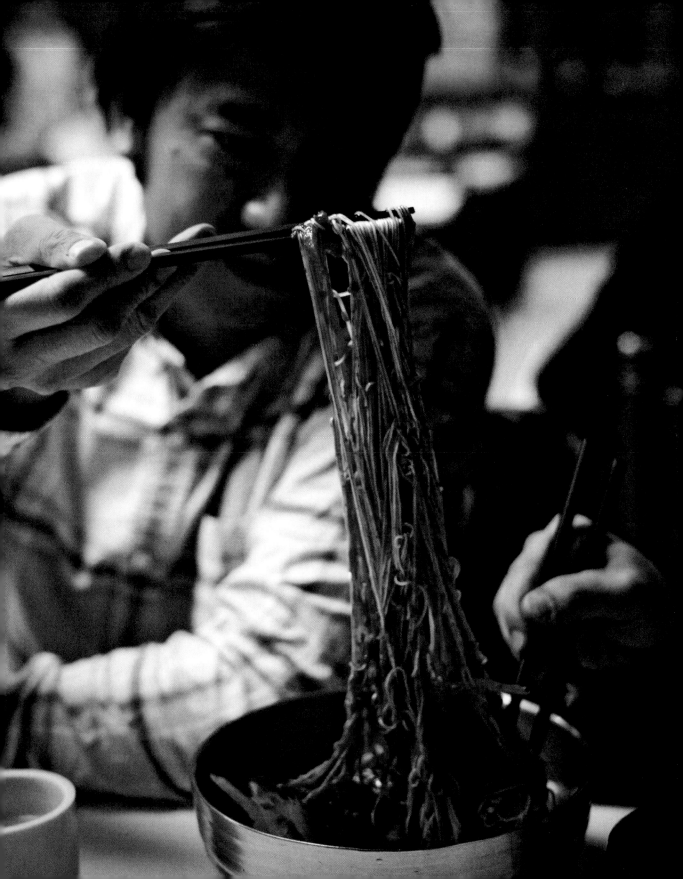

1. **MAKE THE SAUCE:** Combine ingredients in a bowl. Mix well until it all . . . becomes one! (*Ahhhhhhhhhhhhhhhhhhhhhh!*) Cover and refrigerate.
2. Then get ready to eat some cold noodle deliciousness . . . and bring a pot of water to boil over high heat! While waiting for that rolling boil, prepare an ice water bath in a bowl.
3. Once you have a rolling boil, drop in noodles and cook until they're al dente. Once they're done, remove from pot, shake off excess water, and immediately shock in ice water bath for 2 minutes. Remove, shake off excess water, then transfer to a mixing bowl.

   Add sauce and mix. Once noodles are thoroughly covered, arrange in a bowl and garnish with pear, cucumber, scallions, watermelon, pickled watermelon radish, and sesame seeds, along with your Soft-Boiled Egg, yolk facing up . . . yummmmmmers!

DAN DAN NOODLES/MIEN

Dan dan mien is a classic Szechuan dish made with the unique mouth-numbing Szechuan pepper corns. It's so flavorful. It's delicious. It's the most sent back dish at Button Mash, and one of the most loved ones as well. Numbing sensations ain't for everyone.

2–4 SERVINGS

SAUCE:

¼ cup Superconcentrated Cantonese Chicken Stock (page 256)

2 tablespoons light soy sauce

½ tablespoon Chinese sesame paste

1 tablespoon Chinkiang brand vinegar

3 tablespoons chili oil

2 teaspoons sesame oil

1½ teaspoons sugar

2 teaspoons Szechuan/Sichuan red pepper corns, dry roasted

NOODLES:

2 tablespoons minced garlic

1 teaspoon minced ginger

3 tablespoons chopped scallions

2 tablespoons Szechuan/Sichuan preserved vegetables *

½ pounds ground pork

1 tablespoon Chinese cooking wine

½ teaspoon kosher salt

8 ounces fresh ramen noodles or 11 ounces dry noodles (refer to Garlic Noodle recipe, page 25, for notes, options, and thoughts on other noodles)

Cilantro, for garnish

Peanuts, coarsely chopped, for garnish

Crispy shallots, for garnish

Black pepper, freshly cracked, for garnish

Pickled Mustard Greens, (page 247), for garnish

* Preserved = pickled, and they're pretty standard at most Asian stores. Play around with different ones to figure out the ones you like best (especially for this dish)

BALLS OUT

40–80 SERVINGS

SAUCE:

5 cups Superconcentrated Cantonese Chicken Stock (page 256)

2½ cups light soy sauce

10 tablespoons Chinese sesame paste

1¼ cups Chinkiang brand vinegar

3¾ cups chili oil

¾ cups plus 1⅓ tablespoons sesame oil

10 tablespoons sugar

¾ cups plus 1⅓ tablespoons Szechuan/Sichuan red pepper corns, dry roasted

NOODLES:

2½ cups minced garlic

6⅔ tablespoons minced ginger

3¾ cups chopped scallions

2½ cups Szechuan/Sichuan preserved vegetables *

10 pounds ground pork

1¼ cups Chinese cooking wine

3⅓ tablespoons kosher salt

10 pounds fresh ramen noodles or 13¾ pounds dry noodles (refer to Garlic Noodle recipe, page 25, for notes, options, and thoughts on other noodles)

1. **FOR THE (LOVE OF) SAUCE:** Combine all sauce ingredients in a bowl. Mix well. Set aside.

2. **NOODLES FOR THE WIN:** Set up an ice bath in a bowl large enough to hold the noodles in.

3. Heat up a pot of 2-inches of water until you achieve a rolling boil. Drop noodles in and time. (Refer to the Garlic Noodle [Make-Out Noodles], to advise on best al dente times.)

4. Then remove noodles from pot, shake off excess and shock noodles in ice bath for 2 minutes. Remove, shake of excess, and transfer noodles to serving bowl. Set aside.

5. Heat up a pan with a little bit of oil over medium heat, and sauté garlic, ginger, scallions, and preserved vegetables together until fragrant. Then add pork and stir-fry while breaking apart until it is a tad crispy and no longer pink.

   Next add Chinese wine and scrape up all the bits to deglaze the pan. Season with salt. Remove from heat, transfer to bowl of noodles. Top meat with ¼ cup of your recently mixed sauce. Garnish with scallions, peanuts, shallots, black pepper, and pickled mustard greens on the side. Mix, and enjoy the numbing flavors . . . unless your mouth is so numb that it reminds you of being in a dentist's chair, then slow down and enjoy life a little bit more maybe.

BANH BEO (AKA STEAMED VIETNAMESE RICE CREPE)

This is one of my favoritest things EVAR in the world, which I'm realizing I say for many of these dishes. When I was a kid, my parents stocked shitloads of aluminum steamers in our garage, and an even larger shitload of baby food tops, which we used to make ALL the *banh beo* in. They hosted parties where all they and their friends would do was eat hundreds of these and drink BEER! How cool were my parents, huh? Beer and *banh beo* ragers—that sounds like the life to me.

BALLS OUT
40–80 SERVINGS

10 cups rice flour

10 tablespoons tapioca starch

5 quarts water

1⅔ tablespoons kosher salt

3⅓ tablespoons chicken bouillon

3⅓ tablespoons cooking oil

2–4 SERVINGS

1 cup rice flour

1 tablespoon tapioca starch

2 cups water

½ teaspoon kosher salt

1 teaspoon chicken bouillon

1 teaspoon cooking oil

GARNISH:

Coco Rice Vietnamese Fish Sauce (page 240)

Pork rinds

Dried shrimp (tiny)

Mint chiffonade

Thai chilies, finely chopped

Mung beans (optional)

Scallion Oil (optional; check Grilled Fish Heads and Tails recipe, page 128, to make it)

1. Combine rice flour, tapioca starch, water, salt, and chicken bouillon in a bowl. Stir until a singular liquid consistency forms. Let it settle. The water will separate to the top.

2. Once the top layer of water is clear, carefully pour the water out into a measuring cup. Take note of the exact measurement, dispose of water, replace with the same amount of new water, and pour back into the original batter bowl. Add oil, but don't stir. Set aside for at least 15 minutes or longer—as long as the batter has time to settle and the new top water layer is clear again—before cooking.

3. **STEAMING THE BANH BEO:** If you're Asian fancy and have a multitiered steamer to make all sorts of *banh beo*, dim sum, steamed buns, and all that jazz, you're a step ahead of most people . . . possibly in life, but mainly in steaming food. (Please invite me over!)

4. If you don't have that, now's the time to get creative and understand how to use a steamer and what you need from it. We hope this hack and explanation will lead you down the path of a setup that will work

the same way to achieve the *banh beo* rager we all want to get to.

5. The main thing to understand about a steamer is that you need to be able to enclose it so you can engulf in steam whatever it is you're steaming!

6. The best way to approach this is to use a pot that already has an existing cover. Find a (nonplastic) bowl large and sturdy enough to hold up a (also nonplastic) plate on top of it but small enough to fit inside the pot. Place the bowl in the pot. Fill the bowl with water to weigh it down. Then fill the pot with enough water to sit below the top rim of the bowl. The bowl should remain still in the pot; it shouldn't float. This might get tricky, so you may want to interchange the step of the water in the bowl and pot until you can get the bowl to sit still in your pot filled with water.

7. Place a suitable plate on top of the bowl. You still with me? Bueller?

8. This is your steamer . . . or whatever better version you create instead with the same principles kept in mind.

9. Regarding the individual *banh beo*, if you can find one, you can use a fancy aluminum steam dish tray thing made specifically for steaming that accommodates ten to twelve *banh beo* at a time. This will replace the plate in the above hack.

10. Or you can do it like my 'rents did and use baby food tops as your steam dish of choice, or shallow Asian sauce dipping dishes, which are about 2 to 3 inches in diameter, as individual steam dishes on top of the plate.

11. Since you got all those hacks, let's proceed, shall we?

12. If you haven't already, fill steamer with enough water to stay at a constant rolling boil to steam all or as much of the *banh beo* as possible. The water shouldn't ever completely evaporate in this process. Cover and bring water to rolling boil over high heat.

13. While waiting for the water to boil, organize everything (batter, steaming dishes, ladles, etc.) into a station as close to the steamer and as logically as possible (aka *mise en place* aka "everything in its place" . . . Yay!). This is helpful so you aren't fumbling around and helps you keep a calm head while attacking this beautiful beast of a dish.

14. Before each round of cooking, lightly line each steam dish with oil either with a brush or pan spray. This will make it much easier to

remove each *banh beo* (especially if you're starting an illegal restaurant in your apartment. Every extra minute counts!).

15. Ladle batter into steam dishes, stirring batter before each new scoop. If you're using the makeshift steamer, I recommend leaving the plate inside the pot all the time, placing/removing the steam dishes by hand (with gloves), unless you have a consistently safe way to remove and place the plate back in. All joking aside, please be very careful and don't burn yourself.

16. Cover and steam for 2–3 minutes; adjust time depending on results. If the *banh beo* are still watery, they need to steam longer; if they're rubbery, they need to steam for a shorter amount of time. The final product should be slightly flimsy, a little bit slippery, lightly chewy, and act as a delicious device with which you can enjoy all the toppings.

17. Remove steam dishes from pot, check the pot's water level, and if you still have more *banh beo* to steam, pour in more water if it's running low. Cover the pot to keep the rolling boil going until the next round. Allow the *banh beo* dishes to cool for a minute or two out of the steamer. Repeat until batter is all used (though you can refrigerate unused batter and use it later).

18. Once *banh beo* dishes are cooled down, garnish *banh beo* individually with fish sauce, pork rinds, dried shrimp, mint, Thai chilies, and mung bean (my least liked, though traditional, garnish). Spoon out *banh beo* to eat. Or, scoop out *banh beo* prior to garnishing, then lay them down overlapping one another on a plate. Use the same garnishes, and enjoy by yourself or family style. Don't worry; Vietnamese people eat it both ways.

Enjoy the *banh beo* rager, y'all!

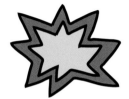

POPIAH (AKA BO BIA)

So THIS dish exists in so many different forms in so many different neighboring countries with so many different variations on the name that even we debated about which name to use. Ultimately, we chose *popiah* (pronounced "Bo-BEE-a"). No matter how you say it, this dish is a fresh vegetarian—always vegetarian—spring roll common in Southeast Asia.

2–4 SERVINGS

Soy Bean Jicama
(page 187)

French/Green/Long
Beans (page 187)

Curry Tofu "Fries"
(page 190)

Good Ol' Omelet
(page 190)

Hoisin Peanut Dipping
Sauce (page 191)

Pickled Kohlrabi
(page 246)

Persian cucumbers,
julienned

Carrots, julienned

Rice paper *

* We use rice paper
instead of the chewy

freshly made popiah
wrapper, which is
fantastic if you haven't
had it. You can look up
tons of YouTube videos
on how to make it and
what it looks like.

1. We do this dish a little bit differently from what's traditional. But isn't that part of the fun? We also want to give you the full Button Mash experience—as a family-style wrap-it-yourself affair.

2. Every major affair component is served in its own separate bowls: jicama, beans, tofu, egg, peanut sauce, Pickled Kohlrabi, cucumbers, carrots, and rice paper.

3. For the rice paper, you can soften it either using a bowl of warm water or cold water (if you're a wrapping n00b and need slower softening time to figure out how you're gonna wrap these suckers), OR, if you're an uber-pro like my mother-in-law, who brought back from Vietnam those vertical rice paper holders and dipping stands, using one of those. (You can find them online, and we use them at Button Mash—seriously one of the best space-saving inventions ever!)

4. Gather friends and family and wrap away at your very own *popiah*-wrapping festival.

    BUT if you're a considerate host and know that most of your guests don't like doing all that, cut the beans into 1-inch pieces, and then throw ALL the major components into a big bowl (like in Thi's family's kitchen), hand mix all of it together, and premake as many rolls as you can—*then* have a *popiah*-eating festival wherever you POPIIIIIIIIIIIIIIIIIIIIIIIAH!

SOY BEAN JICAMA

2–4 SERVINGS

5 shallots, peeled and sliced

½ tablespoon soybean sauce (but the consistency is really like a paste, FYI)

½ pound jicama, peeled and julienned

½ cup water

½ tablespoon sugar

½ tablespoon dark soy sauce

½ tablespoon sugar

Kosher salt

BALLS OUT
40–80 SERVINGS

20 shallots, peeled and sliced

10 tablespoons soybean sauce

10 pounds jicama, peeled and julienned

10 cups water

10 tablespoons sugar

10 tablespoons dark soy sauce

10 tablespoons sugar

Kosher salt

In a pan/wok, over medium heat, add the shallots, and cook until golden: Mix in the pasty soybean sauce and stir frequently until the mixture is fragrant.

Toss in the jicama, stirring quickly, then add water, sugar, and dark soy sauce. Bring the mixture to a boil and let simmer for 10 minutes, or until jicama softens but still retains its crunch. It should adopt some of the soybean color while keeping a hint of the original white color as well. Season with additional sugar and salt, if necessary. It should taste savory with some sweetness.

FRENCH/GREEN/ LONG BEANS

2–4 SERVINGS

3½ ounces French long beans, cut into 3-inch segments *

2 shallots, peeled and sliced

1 teaspoon finely chopped garlic

2 pinches kosher salt

2 pinches mushroom bouillon

2 pinches sugar

* Aka *haricot vert,* aka Harry-Co-Ver-T . . . but not really.

BALLS OUT
40–80 SERVINGS

4⅓ pounds French long beans, cut into 3-inch segments *

40 shallots, peeled and sliced

6⅔ tablespoons finely chopped garlic

2½ teaspoons kosher salt

2½ teaspoons mushroom bouillon

2½ teaspoons sugar

1. Bring a pot of salted water to a boil over high heat. Prepare an ice water bath to hold the beans after they're cooked.
2. When the water reaches a rolling boil, add beans and cook for 2 minutes, then remove from pot and shock in ice water to retain the crunchy texture of the beans.
3. In a pan, add some oil over medium heat. Add shallots and cook until light golden in color, then garlic. Give it a quick stir. Increase heat to high, add beans, and stir-fry 2–3 minutes. Season with salt, mushroom bouillon, and sugar.

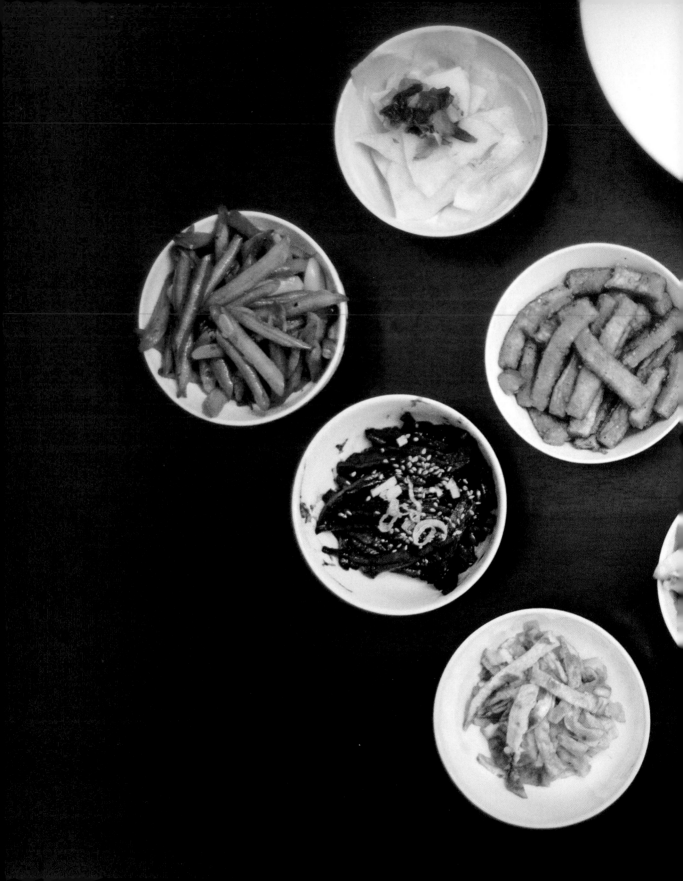

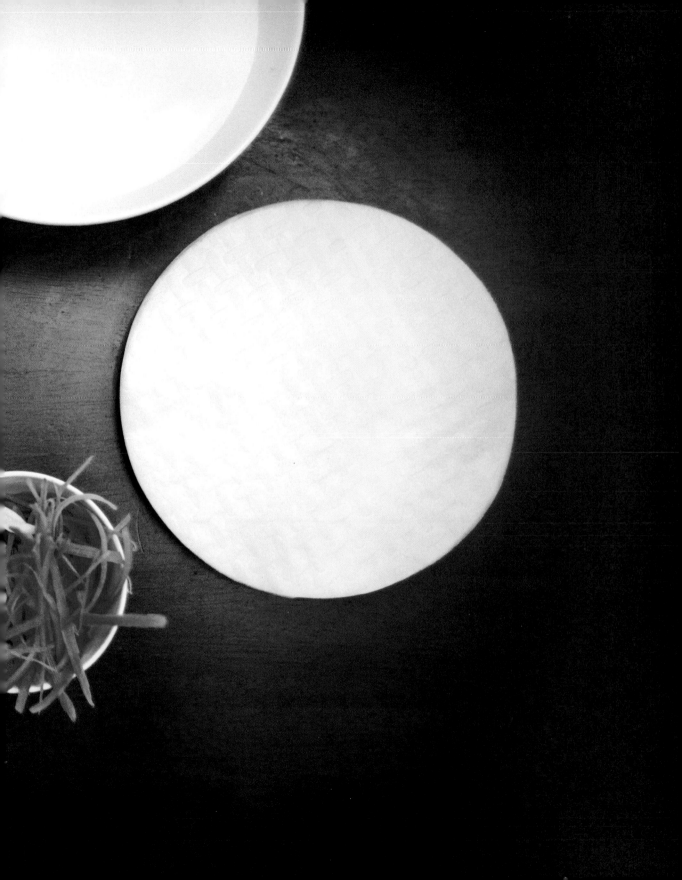

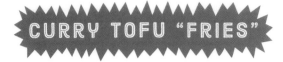

CURRY TOFU "FRIES"

9½ ounces (half a 19-ounce box) firm tofu*

1 cup cornstarch

½ tablespoon kosher salt

1 tablespoon curry powder

½ teaspoon ground white pepper

1 tablespoon mushroom bouillon

* Use the other half of the tofu to make Lemongrass Tofu or even Crispy Tofu Balls. The world of tofu is yours for the takin', friends!

BALLS OUT
40–80 SERVINGS

190 ounces (10 19-ounce boxes) firm tofu*

5 quarts cornstarch

10 tablespoons kosher salt

1¼ cups curry powder

6⅔ tablespoons ground white pepper

1¼ cups mushroom bouillon

1. Heat a pot with 1 inch oil to 350°F over medium-high heat. While waiting for the oil to heat, cut tofu blocks into "fries" a little bit larger than McDonald's french fries.

2. Season cornstarch with salt, curry powder, white pepper, and mushroom bouillon in a bowl. Mix in very well. Full-coat tofu fries with cornstarch mix, shake off excess.

   When oil reaches temperature, fry tofu fries until golden in color and crispy in texture. Remove from oil, shake off excess, and serve.

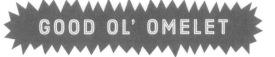

GOOD OL' OMELET

2 large eggs

2 pinches kosher salt

2 pinches sugar

1 pinch ground black pepper

BALLS OUT
40–80 SERVINGS

40 large eggs

2½ teaspoons kosher salt

2½ teaspoons sugar

1¼ teaspoon black pepper

1. Crack eggs into a bowl and beat lightly. Add salt, sugar, and pepper.

2. Heat a pan over medium heat with some cooking oil. Pour eggs in pan, and swirl mixture around the pan making sure egg distributes evenly. Cook without disturbing the egg for about 1–2 minutes, or until the egg is solid enough to check the underside. Flip half the egg over the other half, or flip the entire omelet to cook through for 1 minute. Do not brown. Remove from heat and pat dry excess oil. Then julienne omelet, and set aside in a bowl.

   If you want to go all French-style omelet, roll the omelet from one side of the pan to the other while reducing the heat to get the perfect roll. It'll come out really pretty, except you'll probably want to cook the egg through (for this recipe) or else it'll be a runny mess when trying to julienne.

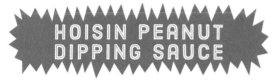

HOISIN PEANUT DIPPING SAUCE

2–4 SERVINGS

¼ cup crunchy peanut butter

2 tablespoons hoisin sauce

1 tablespoon rice vinegar

2 teaspoons minced garlic

2 teaspoons chili paste (aka *sambal oelek*)

5 tablespoons water

BALLS OUT

40–80 SERVINGS

5 cups crunchy peanut butter

2⅓ cups plus 2 tablespoons hoisin sauce

1¼ cups rice vinegar

¾ cup minced garlic

¾ cup chili paste (aka *sambal oelek*)

6 cups plus 2 tablespoons water

Combine ingredients in a pot over medium-low heat. Mix well. Consistency should be thick and viscous. If it's runny, lower or remove from heat while mixing until it gets thicker. Warm up sauce on low heat when ready to serve. Voilà— dip! ☺

My favorite *popiah* memory was the first time I hung out with all of Thi's huge extended family in San Francisco in the Richmond district (a couple blocks south of Clement if you want to get real specific and real Cantonese-Chinese up in dis house). It was one of those romantically brisk and chill San Francisco winter days when everyone mostly just wanted to stay warm inside. And inside the kitchen—with all the aunties cooking, all the cousins running around causing havoc, all the uncles babbling about whatever uncles babble about, and Thi's recently widowed grandmother just taking it all in and laughing—was this HUGE bowl of *popiah* mix. Then all the aunts began rolling the *popiah*. They insisted I eat one, and while I was internally reticent to try, because there was no meat in it whatsoever, I ate it. And I fell in love with the dish, deeper in love with Thi and the package that is her family that came along with her, and back in love with the classic feeling of family and the food that comes with that.

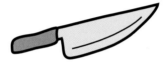

SPAM BRUSSELS SPROUT FRIED RICE

There's a lot of debate about what spiritually and physically makes a great fried rice and some other BS. But the real true winning-est answer known by about every Asian on planet Earth this side of the solar system and in a galaxy known to some as the Milky Way: It's SPAM. End of debate. I won't accept any other sides to this argument, mainly because I'll be too busy stuffing my face with Spam Brussels Sprout Fried Rice.

BALLS OUT
40–80 SERVINGS

12½ ounces Brussels sprouts

1½ cups brown sugar

6¼ pounds Spam, sliced ¾-inch thick

50 large eggs

1½ cups coarsely chopped garlic

6¼ cups shredded carrots

25 serrano chili peppers

25 quarts cooked, day-old jasmine rice *

8⅓ tablespoons chicken bouillon

8⅓ tablespoons white pepper†

8⅓ tablespoons kosher salt

8⅓ tablespoons sugar

12½ cups chopped cilantro, plus additional for garnish

2–4 SERVINGS

½ ounce (small handful) Brussels sprouts, halved

1 tablespoon brown sugar

4 ounces Spam, sliced ¾-inch thick

2 large eggs

1 tablespoon coarsely chopped garlic

¼ cup shredded carrots

1 serrano chili pepper

4 cups cooked, day-old jasmine rice*

1 teaspoon chicken bouillon

1 teaspoon white pepper†

1 teaspoon kosher salt

1 teaspoon sugar

½ cup chopped cilantro, plus additional for garnish

* If you don't have any jasmine rice, any long-grain rice will do. BUT if you're using medium, short, or, heaven forbid, my favorite Vietnamese breakfast of a lifetime, broken (jasmine) rice, fried rice becomes a bit harder to accomplish. It's gonna be different, but whatevs—have at it, and Instagram it with the hashtag #stuffitSK.

† Black pepper is NOT the same as white pepper—so get white pepper if you can. It's REALLY different. I PROMISE.

1. Let's start with caramelizing the Brussels by adding some oil to a pan on high heat. Then throwing in the Brussels once the oil starts to smoke just a tad, and adding brown sugar and stir-frying for 2–3 minutes until they get a good golden caramel color with some char on the Brussels as well. Remove from heat, set Brussels aside in a bowl, and clean pan so the sugars don't burn the rest of the recipe.

2. Now here's the secret to really getting the flavor and achieving true Spam Karma ("Welcome to karmic Spam enlightenment, my child"): Heat up a pan with some cooking oil to medium-high heat. Once the pan's hot, sear slices of gelatinous Spam amazingness and watch them turn into tasty swans of *sabor* ("flavor" in Spanish). Don't flip

over until you get a nice char on one side; then flip and sear the other. Remove from pan (but don't clean the pan yet). Cut your Spam-mini-steaks into ¾-inch cubes. Try the crustiest one to see what all the crispy Spamy enlightenment fuss is all about.

3. Whisk the eggs in a bowl, add a dash of salt, and set aside.

4. In the Spam-flavored pan, add 1 tablespoon cooking oil on high heat. Once the pan is hot, add the garlic, carrots, and serranos to the pan individually in that order and sauté until each is lightly browned before adding the next. Set aside together in a bowl.

5. Keep pan on high heat; add and cook eggs for 15–20 seconds. Eggs should be runny. Set aside back in original bowl.

6. Add a little bit more oil and the day-old cooked rice. Mix in until you get good color on the rice, breaking all the clumps apart. Be careful not to dry out. If you do, add less than a tablespoon more oil and stir-fry rice again.

7. Add sautéed garlic, carrots, and serranos. Mix in to rice. Decrease to medium heat and add chicken bouillon, white pepper, salt, and sugar. Mix well.

8. Next, add Spam and Brussels sprouts, while constantly mixing and moving the rice around the pan. Add eggs and mix into rice.

9. Add cilantro, then quickly mix for 5–10 seconds. Remove pan from heat.

Plate in a nice big family-style bowl, garnish with a little more cilantro, and share or eat by yourself while you sit in front of your TV watching *Nashville* and *Empire* (they're my TV yin and yang). Enjoy eating . . . and the spectacular TV catfights in store for you!

GALANGAL CHICKEN FRIED RICE

After our Kickstarter campaign to raise $500k failed, we had a lot of leftover food that we took home because (1) we had it, (2) waste is my biggest pet peeve, and (3) we didn't have a backup plan except for the fact that we could live off of our leftovers for a long time. Out of hunger and necessity, we used one of those dishes, unwrapped Pandan/Galangal Chicken, which we always thought would be a universally delicious dish, to make fried rice. Eventually it became part of our fried rice starting lineup for Button Mash, too. I'm starting to see a common theme of necessity leading to creativity with us . . . weird! (and delish☺).

2–4 SERVINGS

2 large eggs

5½ ounces Pandan/Galangal Chicken (page 52); uncooked and not wrapped (DELICIOUS!)

¼ cup medium dice yellow or white onion

¼ cup medium dice red bell peppers

NO GARLIC!

4 cups cooked, day-old jasmine rice

1 teaspoon mushroom bouillon

1 teaspoon kosher salt

1 teaspoon sugar

¼ cup Chinese dark soy sauce

Scallions, chopped, for garnish

Cilantro, chopped, for garnish

BALLS OUT
40–80 SERVINGS

50 large eggs

8⅔ pounds Pandan/Galangal Chicken, uncooked and not wrapped

6¼ cups medium dice yellow or white onion

6¼ cups medium dice red bell peppers

NO GARLIC!

25 quarts cooked, day-old jasmine rice

8⅓ tablespoons mushroom bouillon

8⅓ tablespoons kosher salt

8⅓ tablespoons cups sugar

6¼ cups Chinese dark soy sauce

1. Whisk eggs in a bowl, add a dash of salt, and set aside.

2. Heat a pan/wok on high heat with a little bit of oil. Once it's blistering like the sun (or as hot as your stove will get), sauté chicken for 4–5 minutes until it's nicely browned and fully cooked through. Transfer to a bowl and set aside.

3. Add 1 tablespoon cooking oil to the same pan on high heat. Once the pan is hot, sauté the following ingredients one by one until each is lightly browned before adding the next, in this order: onions, and bell peppers. Once done, set aside in a bowl.

4. Keep pan on high heat, add and cook eggs for 15–20 seconds. Eggs should still be runny. Set aside in original bowl.

5. Keeping a high heat, add a little more oil and day-old cooked rice. Mix until you get good color on the rice, breaking all the clumps

apart. Be careful not to dry out. If you do, add less than a tablespoon more oil and stir-fry rice again.

6. Add sautéed onions and bell peppers. Mix in. Decrease to medium heat and add mushroom bouillon, salt, and sugar. Mix well.

7. Add dark soy sauce and mix thoroughly.

8. Add chicken while constantly stirring and moving the rice around the pan. Then add the runny eggs. Mix into rice.

Remove pan from heat immediately. Plate in a nice big family-style bowl, garnish with scallions and cilantro, and share.

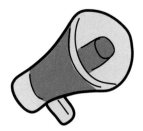

SHRIMP AND GRILLED PINEAPPLE FRIED RICE

There are a few foods I can't stand and can't make myself eat, like cantaloupe.

The other: bean sprouts. I don't like 'em! I know I'm Asian, but I don't like 'em cooked, and I don't like 'em raw. But for some reason this fried rice is so delectable that I don't mind 'em in this. And I can't even remember where the combination of the shrimp and grilled pineapple came from, but wherever it came from, it's delish and one of the fried rice trifecta at Button Mash . . . and I'm downright cool with that. ☺

2–4 SERVINGS

2 large eggs

¼ pound uncooked, head-off, tail-off, deveined (U60–80) shrimp

1 tablespoon coarsely chopped garlic

¼ cup medium dice yellow or white onions

¼ cup shredded carrots

¼ cup bean sprouts

4 cups cooked, day-old jasmine rice

1 teaspoon mushroom bouillon

1 teaspoon kosher salt

1 pinch ground white pepper

1 teaspoon sugar

¼ cup Chinese light soy sauce

1 red Fresno chili, sliced into rings

¼ cup medium dice grilled pineapples

¼ cup chopped scallions, plus additional for garnish

5 sprigs cilantro, chopped, plus additional for garnish

BALLS OUT
40–80 SERVINGS

50 large eggs

6¼ pounds uncooked, head-off, tail-off, deveined (U60–80) shrimp

1½ cups coarsely chopped garlic

6¼ cups medium dice yellow or white onions

6¼ cups shredded carrots

6¼ cups bean sprouts

25 quarts cooked, day-old jasmine rice

8⅓ tablespoons mushroom bouillon

8⅓ tablespoons kosher salt

1½ teaspoons white pepper

8⅓ tablespoons sugar

6¼ cups Chinese light soy sauce

25 red Fresno chilies, sliced into rings

6¼ cups medium dice grilled pineapples

6¼ cups chopped scallions, plus additional for garnish

1 bunch cilantro, chopped, plus additional for garnish

1. Whisk eggs in a bowl, add a dash of salt, and set aside.
2. Heat a pan/wok on high heat with a little bit of oil. Sauté shrimp for 3–4 minutes, stopping short of cooking them all the way through. Transfer shrimp to a bowl and set aside.
3. In the shrimpy flavored pan, add 1 tablespoon cooking oil on high heat. Once the pan is hot, sauté garlic, onions, carrots, and bean sprouts one by one in that order, browning each one lightly before adding the next. Set aside in a bowl.
4. Keep pan on high heat, add and cook eggs for 15–20 seconds. Eggs should be runny. Set aside in bowl.
5. Keeping a high heat, add a little bit more oil and the day-old cooked rice. Mix until you get good color on the rice, breaking all the clumps apart. Be careful not to dry out. If you do, add less than a tablespoon more oil and stir-fry rice again.
6. Add sautéed garlic, onions, carrots, and bean sprouts. Mix in. Lower to medium heat and add mushroom bouillon, salt, white pepper, and sugar. Mix in well.
7. Add light soy sauce, and mix thoroughly.
8. Add shrimp and Fresno chilies while constantly mixing and moving the rice around the pan. Stir-fry for a minute to cook the shrimp through. Then add in the runny eggs, and mix with rice.
9. Add pineapples, scallions, and cilantro. Give all a quick toss, then immediately remove from heat.

Plate in a nice big family-style bowl, garnish with scallions and cilantro, and share or eat by yourself while reminiscing about how the kids movies of the 1980s, like *The Goonies, E.T.,* and *The NeverEnding Story,* were so awesome.

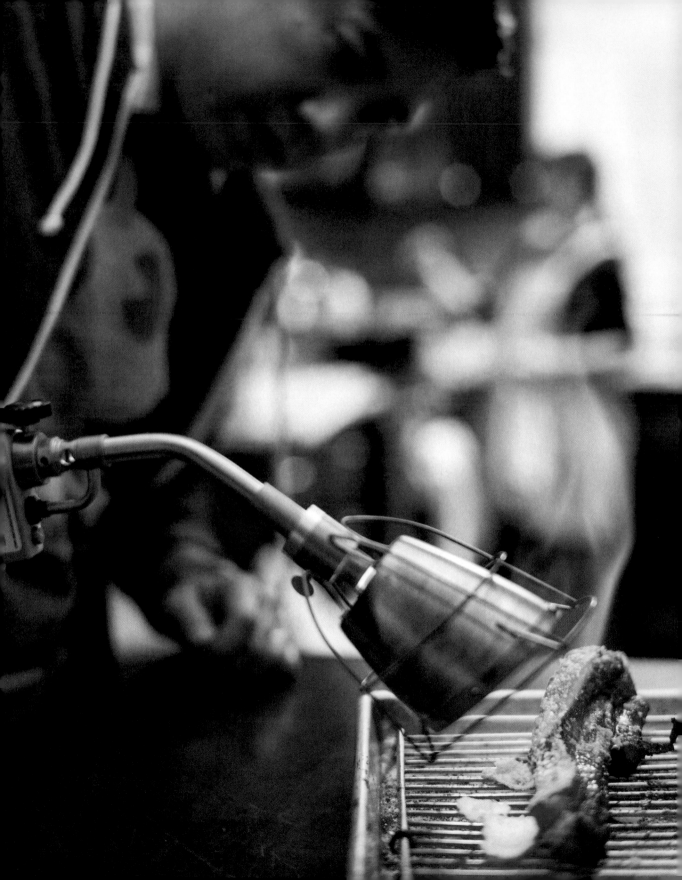

ROAST PORK BELLY

I don't know if eating meat gets any better than this, especially when that skin is crunch-ay! The best compliment (aka Yelp review) we often get about this dish is people telling us it tastes EXACTLY like we picked it up from an old-school Chinese BBQ spot. And that's exactly what we're going for: classic, crunchy, succulent . . . damn good. Thanks for that "tip" anonymous (1-star) reviewer(s)!

BALLS OUT
40–80 SERVINGS

10 pounds skin-on pork belly*

3⅓ teaspoons five-spice powder

6⅔ teaspoons onion powder

6⅔ teaspoons garlic powder

6⅔ teaspoons light soy sauce

6⅔ teaspoons plus 2¼ cup kosher salt

2–4 SERVINGS

1½ pounds skin-on pork belly*

½ teaspoon five-spice powder

1 teaspoon onion powder

1 teaspoon garlic powder

1 teaspoon light soy sauce

1 teaspoon plus ⅓ cup kosher salt

* Recipe adjustment advice: Your pork belly probably won't weigh exactly 1½ pounds, which is cool. Divide the weight (in pounds) of your pork belly (let's call that x) by 1½ pounds, the weight our recipe calls for, or "$x \div 1.5$," to be exact. That generates your numeric ratio, then multiply that ratio individually with the rest of the ingredients to get the exact measurement adjustments you need. #mathRULES!

1. Wash pork belly under cool running water. Pat dry.
2. Combine five-spice, onion powder, and garlic powder in a small bowl; mix and use it all to dry rub only the entirety of the exposed meat (non-skin) sides. Next rub soy sauce on the exposed meat sides of the pork belly as well. (Do not take a shortcut and combine the soy sauce with the dry ingredients in this recipe, this was written like that intentionally . . . thank you!)
3. Set meat-side down over a baking sheet on a cooking rack. Next, rub 1 teaspoon salt onto skin side of the pork.
4. Refrigerate, uncovered, for 3 days (yup, *72 hours*) to cure for the absolute best flavor.
5. When ready to cook: Remove pork from fridge and let it come to room temperature. Preheat oven to 350°F.
6. Set oven rack between the highest and middle rows. Line a roasting or baking pan with foil. Pat dry the skin-sides of the pork belly with a paper towel, then use the remaining salt to cover the skin completely with

a thick layer. Lay pork on a wire rack on top of the foil. While the pork belly cooks, delicious pork drippings will drip onto the foil. Get ready!

7. Make sure the skin-side is level or it will not crackle as evenly later on (and you know you want it . . . at least *I* do). If it's not level, use something oven-safe to prop it up to keep it completely level.

8. Bake for 50–55 minutes, or until internal temperature (of your pork belly) reaches 145°F at the center-most point and the salt forms a uniform crust across the skin.

9. Remove pork from oven, then increase temperature to 400°F.

10. Remove salt crust (which can sometimes be removed in one piece) and save for fried rice or other porkilicious creations. Scrape off excess salt and pat skin-side dry with a dry towel. Be sure not to dispose of the drippings.

11. Remove wire rack and keep foil in place and then wrap only the sides of pork and drippings in foil with skin-side exposed.

12. Once oven temperature reaches 400°F, place foil-wrapped pork belly back into oven. Bake for 20–25 minutes, or until bubbles start to visibly form on skin.

13. Remove from oven.

14. If the broiler is part of the main oven, relocate the oven rack to the middle shelf. Set broiler on low for 25–30 minutes, or until you get the desired crispy bubbling.

15. If the broiler is located underneath the oven, set the broiler rack to the lowest possible level, then broil on low. Turn off main oven (if it doesn't turn off the broiler), then move baking sheet from oven to broiler. Broil pork for 5–10 minutes, or until you get the desired crispy bubbling.

16. Watch pork closely to prevent burning or uneven bubbling—especially with broilers underneath the oven. If the pork is bubbling unevenly, shift the pork belly toward the point where the broiler flame seems to produce the most even bubbling. Don't be afraid of the fire—get to know your oven! (If you have a fancy blowtorch-like Searzall [we're guilty; we have one], you don't need to do any of this and can use that to carefully bubble up the skin.)

17. Once the pork is bubbled evenly, remove from oven; let sit 10 minutes before serving. Save drippings from the foil for simple dipping, for a more complicated porky dip, or for fried rice.

When carving, cut skin-side down, and plate as an individual entree, over rice, in a *banh mi*, as a fun afternoon snack, or quite possibly make Roast Pork Belly XO Fried Rice!

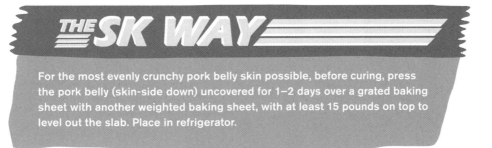

THE SK WAY

For the most evenly crunchy pork belly skin possible, before curing, press the pork belly (skin-side down) uncovered for 1–2 days over a grated baking sheet with another weighted baking sheet, with at least 15 pounds on top to level out the slab. Place in refrigerator.

ROAST PORK BELLY XO FRIED RICE

What's better than fried rice? NOTHING, except maybe Roast Pork Belly XO Fried Rice made with those amazing Roast Pork Belly drippings. XO does not, in this case, refer to cognac. Instead, it's a sauce composed of dried scallops, dried shrimp, pepper, and cured ham all aged together to bring out an extra-savory-not-easily-replicable flavor.

BALLS OUT
40–80 SERVINGS

7 pounds Roast Pork Belly, (page 199), sliced and cut into slivers

50 large eggs

1½ teaspoons kosher salt

3 cups Roast Pork Belly fat, or any oil/fat

150 pieces crushed garlic

4¾ cups shallots

8⅓ cups fresh corn, off the cob

12½ cups diced bell pepper

25 quarts cooked, loosely packed day-old rice

3 cups chicken bouillon

4⅓ tablespoons black pepper

6¼ teaspoons sugar

1¾ cups XO sauce

2 quarts medium chopped scallions

1½ quarts cilantro, coarsely chopped, for garnish

2–4 SERVINGS

4½ ounces Roast Pork Belly (page 199), sliced and cut into slivers

2 large eggs

Pinch kosher salt

2 tablespoons Roast Pork Belly drippings, or any oil/fat

6 pieces crushed garlic

3 tablespoon shallots

⅓ cup fresh corn, off the cob

½ cup diced bell pepper

4 cups cooked, loosely packed day-old rice

2 teaspoons chicken bouillon

½ teaspoon black pepper

¼ teaspoon sugar

1 heaping tablespoon XO sauce

⅓ cup medium chopped scallions

¼ cup cilantro, coarsely chopped, for garnish

1. Prepare Roast Pork Belly. Set aside.
2. Whisk eggs in a bowl, add salt, then set aside.
3. Heat wok/pan on high heat and add 1 tablespoon pork fat. Sauté one by one, in this order: garlic, shallots, corn, and bell peppers. Lightly brown each before adding the next ingredient. Set aside in a bowl.
4. With wok still on high heat, add eggs and cook for 15–20 seconds. Eggs should still be runny. Set aside in a different bowl.
5. Add remaining pork fat to wok, then cooked rice. Mix until you get good color on the rice, breaking all the clumps apart. Make sure rice is not completely dried out. If it is, add less than a tablespoon pork oil, then stir-fry into the rice.
6. Add sautéed garlic, shallots, corn, and bell peppers. Lower to medium heat and add chicken bouillon, black pepper, and sugar. Mix well.
7. Add XO sauce and mix thoroughly. Taste. It should be lightly savory and peppery, with a hint of sweetness. If you feel it's lacking, season to your liking.

8. Add Roast Pork Belly. If the belly is room temperature or recently roasted, go ahead and mix in eggs. If the belly is cold, stir-fry for at least 1–2 minutes or until the pork is hot to the touch, then mix in eggs.

9. Next, add scallions and mix for 5–10 seconds. Remove pan from heat immediately.

Plate in a nice big family-style bowl to share or eat by yourself while you sit in front of your computer monitor watching the endless hilarity of cats playing pianos . . . but not before you garnish with cilantro.

THE SK WAY

Always keep extra Roast Pork Belly fat handy to add more flavor to dried-out or overcooked fried rice.

THE SK WAY

Day-old rice is THE way make fried rice, period! If it's older than that, it might be too dry, and you will need to add some water to it to remoisten it. BUT it could also be at the point of no return and just be crappy. Be careful.

You can use fresh rice, too, for fried rice, but it'll be much harder to stir-fry (but I know, Japanese fried rice is typically made with fresh rice but that's NOT long grain, it's usually a short grain, which is a different game y'all).

VIETNAMESE MINCED BEEF-TACULAR

Originally concocted during our lunch days, this dish looks like it could be a fried rice, but it's not and it's much more than that. One of our all-time favorite dishes, at Starry Kitchen and at home, it also evolved into our most complicated dish in assembly.

2–4 SERVINGS

2 teaspoons palm coconut sugar or dark brown sugar*

2½ teaspoons fish sauce

½ tablespoon minced lemongrass

4 Thai chilies, stemmed and minced

1 tablespoon finely minced shallots or yellow/white onion

2½ teaspoons coconut cream

¼ tablespoon Thai curry powder

½ pound 80–20 ground chuck

RICE STIR-FRY INGREDIENTS:

2 tablespoons any cooking oil, or if you're making this again and saved that oil, Vietnamese Minced Beef-tacular fat

4 cups cooked, loosely packed day-old rice or fresh steamed rice

1 teaspoon kosher salt

1 teaspoon sugar

1 teaspoon chicken bouillon

1 tablespoon chopped scallions

GARNISH:

½ Persian cucumber, julienned

1 tablespoon finely chopped scallions

1 tablespoon fried shallots

2 large fried eggs, sunny side up, with crispy edges

Mint chiffonade

1 tablespoon chopped roasted peanuts (optional)

Pickled Red Onions (page 249)

2 tablespoons Coco Rico Vietnamese Fish Sauce (page 240), plus additional on the side

Pickled Watermelon Rinds (page 251), on the side

* If the palm sugar is the clumpy kind, blend it in a food processor until it's a near-fine grain.

THE SK WAY

Remember to drain excess Vietnamese Minced Beef-tacular fat regularly while the chuck cooks—and to save that Beef-tacular curry-fied fat for any future use. Like for cooking eggs, FTW!

BALLS OUT

40–80 SERVINGS

1⅔ cups palm coconut sugar or dark brown sugar*

2 cups fish sauce

1⅓ cups minced lemongrass

160 Thai chilies, stemmed and minced

2½ cups finely minced shallots or yellow/white onion

2 cups coconut cream

⅔ cup Thai curry powder

20 pounds 80–20 ground chuck

RICE STIR-FRY INGREDIENTS:

5 cups Vietnamese Minced Beef-tacular fat or any cooking oil

40 quarts cooked, loosely packed day-old rice or fresh steamed rice

¾ cup kosher salt

¾ cup sugar

¾ cup chicken bouillon

2½ cups chopped scallions

GARNISH:

20 Persian cucumbers, julienned

2½ cups finely chopped scallions

2½ cups fried shallots

80 large fried eggs, sunny side up, with crispy edges

2½ cups chopped roasted peanuts (optional)

5 cups Coco Rico Vietnamese Fish Sauce (page 240), plus additional on the side

1. In a pot over low heat, dissolve palm sugar in fish sauce. Remove from heat and transfer to a bowl. Add lemongrass, chilies, onion, coconut cream, and curry to that same bowl. Mix thoroughly. Let cool.

2. Combine marinade with ground chuck and use your hands to mix. (There should be a little bit of yellow color throughout the beef.) Refrigerate for at least 1 hour, though we recommend overnight.

3. Heat pan/wok to high heat, then add 2 tablespoons oil. Toss in rice, break up any clumps, and stir-fry. Add kosher salt, sugar, bouillon, and scallions; mix thoroughly for 2–3 minutes. Taste (often). It should have a little bit of savory flavor. Remove from pan, plate, and set aside.

4. Next, lower to medium-high heat, then add 1 tablespoon cooking oil and marinated ground chuck. Flatten out chuck as much as your cooking surface allows, then let it sit until the bottom turns nice and brown and the edges start to cook through.

5. Next, mince chuck with a spatula or wooden spoon while the chuck continues to cook. If most of the beef is already cooked through, decrease to medium heat while mincing. Cook until all the chuck is only slightly browned and fully cooked through. Remove from heat, plate over rice.

6. Garnish in this order: cucumbers, scallions, fried shallots, eggs, mint, peanuts, and Pickled Red Onions. Top off with Coco Rico Vietnamese Fish Sauce. Serve with a side of extra fish sauce and a side of Pickled Watermelon Rinds.

Devour. Break those yolks. Destroy.

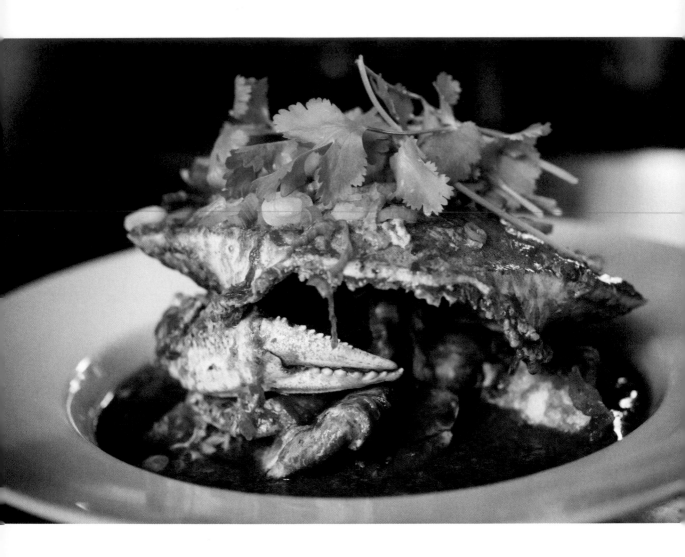

SINGAPOREAN CHILI CRAB

A quick Interwebs search, between watching cats playing piano and cats playing with dogs, revealed ONLY seven other restaurants in all of North America that make this saucy crab dish. Spicy, saucy, and savory—this is a crab dish like NO OTHER. It immediately became Starry Kitchen's OTHER signature dish, along with the infamous Crispy Tofu Balls. People come for our crabs, and our balls . . . and you have fun with the rest.

2–4 SERVINGS

1 fresh Dungeness crab, or equally large and meaty crab *

1 cup cornstarch

AROMATICS:

2 tablespoons minced garlic

2 tablespoons minced shallots

1 tablespoon minced ginger

5 Thai chili peppers, chopped†

1 stalk scallion, cut diagonally

4 cups Chili Crab Sauce (page 212)

2 large eggs

Scallions, for garnish, cut diagonally

Cilantro sprigs, for garnish

5 Buttermilk Beer Beignets (page 213)

* In Singapore, they use the Sri Lankan "Mud" Crab, whose claws are ginormously awesome for eating. If all you can find is frozen crab, be sure to thaw completely before using. But we don't recommend frozen crab; the flavor of the sauce won't be nearly as deep and resonant because frozen crabs are precooked.

† If you want a less spicy dish, here is where you can take some liberties to change this recipe to your liking—but it just ain't as good! Ha-ha.

BALLS OUT
40–80 SERVINGS

20 fresh Dungeness crabs, or equally large and meaty crabs

5 quarts cornstarch

AROMATICS:

2½ cups minced garlic

2½ cups minced shallots

1¼ cups minced ginger

100 Thai chili peppers, chopped

20 stalks scallions, cut diagonally

20 quarts Chili Crab Sauce (page 212)

40 large eggs

1 quart scallions, for garnish, cut diagonally

5 bunches cilantro sprigs, for garnish

100 Buttermilk Beer Beignets (page 213)

1. Clean crab and cut into pieces. If you have never done this before, this might sound easier said than done, but it's not nearly as daunting as it seems.

2. In a debate of "humane" ways of killing crab: the Asian preparation of crab is a near-instant killing of the crab versus the longer and drawn out steaming/boiling method. Additionally, the boiling method tends to result in a much fishier "crabby" flavor, not as fresh tasting as with this method. If you look up videos on YouTube, look up "How to kill a live crab humanely," which will demonstrate this way of breaking down a crab.

3. With that said, I wasn't as prepared in the photograph process, so I'm going to personally walk you through this as the first "Crab Killer" at Starry Kitchen:

4. Quick tips: put crabs in the freezer or refrigerator before breaking down. It will make them sleepy—slow them down very severely. There is also a way one of our cooks, Sean, uncovered on the web to gently pet a soft spot on their shell over and over and they'll start falling asleep. We've seen it. It's crazy, but it takes a lot longer than the freezer method.

5. Next, when you're ready, you're going to need a decently sharp knife for this process or at least one with a sharp tip for this next step: try to grab the crab from the tail end, and flip the crab over, claws and eyes pointing away from you, and so it's belly-side up. If you look at its abdomen right in the center, you'll see a longer triangular lip (top of it pointing away from you) that can actually be lifted up. Until you're comfortable doing it often, you can use the tip of your knife to lift it up, but you'll want to use your hand to quickly just lift up and fold it over completely. The crab will potentially get VERY mad at this point. You've just exposed its most vulnerable spot.

6. Then, this part is simple if you can move quickly: just stab it downward right through that spot that's been exposed until you reach the shell. Hold for about 10–20 seconds. The crab should die almost instantly.

7. Afterwards, line your knife across the middle, and firmly press down and cleave it through the abdomen to cut the crab in half. The crab will snap in half once you come all the way down. You'll also be able to pull the crab by each of its claws, and it'll just come apart.

8. You'll then want to turn each half over, and remove the white gills off of each and dispose.

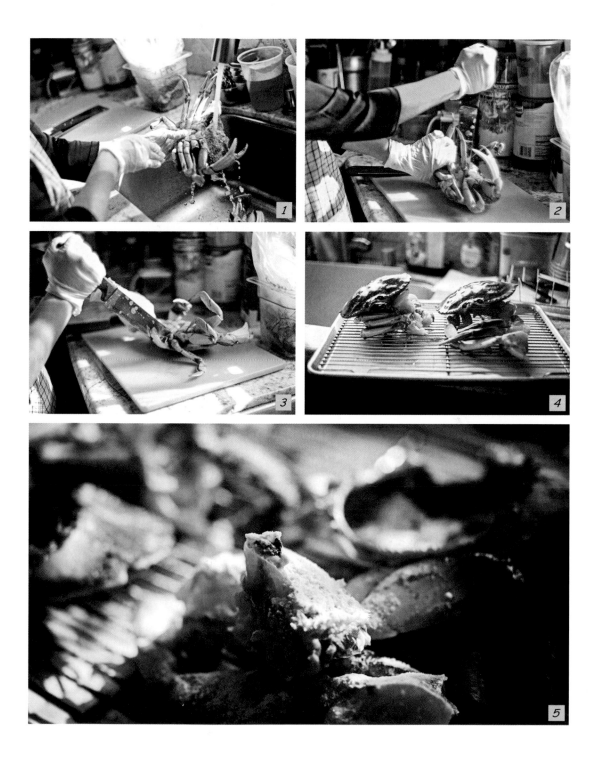

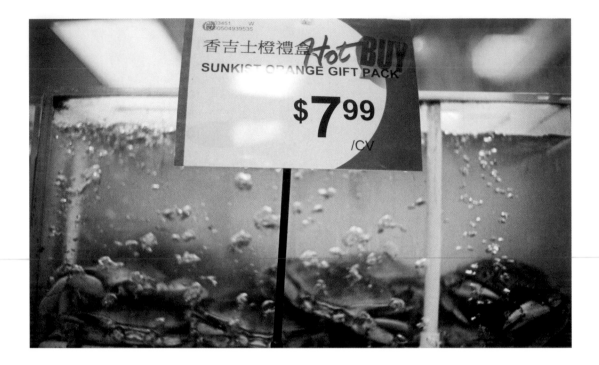

9. Dispose of the lip, and any other loose appendages from the front and back end of the crab.

10. Dispose of the white film and any black matter inside the shell itself, but do not clean out the rest of the shell. That orange part, the coral, the fatty tissue is the MOST coveted part of the crab in Asian households (typically held for the father, no joke). It's like sea urchin/ uni, really rich and very briny . . . and super-awesome to put rice into once it's cooked and scoop it out with. Yummers!

11. Depending on how large your crab is, the two halves of crab legs can be broken into either 2 or 3 sections (there should be a minimum of 2 legs per section) using the same cleaving action as you did to halve the crab.

12. And that's it! (If YouTube, this, and the web doesn't help you feel more comfortable—seriously, feel free to reach out to us: @starrykitchen. This dish is COMPLETELY worth it.)

13. Now clean the crab legs again, then pat dry with paper towels. Put into a big bowl with cornstarch, but make sure to leave enough room to coat crab with starch.

14. Diligently dredge all exposed crab pieces including the coral and head, inside and out, with starch. Next, shake off excess starch, but make sure all of the exposed (non-shelled) parts are covered in starch. This seals in all of the crab's flavors throughout the cooking process. This is especially important if you need to prepare in advance.

15. Fill a wok/pot with 2–3 inches cooking oil, enough to submerge crab pieces, including the head. Heat oil to 350°F over high heat, then carefully fry in batches, arranging crab pieces in a single layer in the oil. Turn over pieces with tongs to fry evenly.

16. When the crab pieces turn red all over and the battered parts are golden, remove and shake the excess oil over your pot. Set aside (we like to set crab on a rack/grate and baking sheet to allow a little bit more oil to drip off). Refrigerate for up to 24 hours.

17. Once you're ready to make your chili crab, heat a wok/pan on high heat and add 1 tablespoon cooking oil per crab. Sauté garlic, shallots, ginger, and chilies until aromatic (enough to make you cough—that's how you know you got the GOOD stuff). Next, add the beautiful monstrosity that is your crab. Stir quickly for 10–15 seconds, then add the Chili Crab Sauce. Cover, cook over high heat, and cook that bad boy (or girl) for 7 minutes.

18. Keep the pan over heat, but remove crab from pan and place on a serving dish. While reconstructing your sea beast, make sure to leave all the sauce in the wok/pan. Crack eggs into the sauce, and quickly mix to fully incorporate them and thicken the sauce. Increase to high heat and reduce sauce to desired thickness. (I like it pretty thick and a little bit gloppy GOOD.)

Once done, remove from heat, and pour sauce all over the crab. Garnish with chopped scallions and cilantro. Serve with Buttermilk Beer Beignets. Break down the crab, sop up all that sauce, and eat like a Singaporean king!

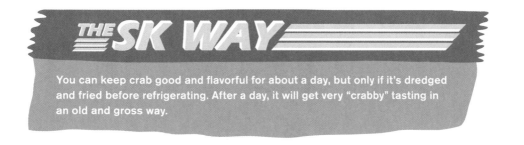

THE SK WAY

You can keep crab good and flavorful for about a day, but only if it's dredged and fried before refrigerating. After a day, it will get very "crabby" tasting in an old and gross way.

CHILI CRAB SAUCE

With this recipe we're giving you the keys to the veritable crabby sauce kingdom. Alter ingredients at your own risk because it took us a LONG time to perfectly balance these flavors!

BALLS OUT
40–80 SERVINGS

15 quarts Superconcentrated Cantonese Chicken Stock, (page 256), hot

5 quarts Hunts brand ketchup*

5 cups light soy sauce

5 cups Lee Kum Kee brand chili garlic sauce

5 cups rice vinegar

5 cups sugar

2–4 SERVINGS

3 cups Superconcentrated Cantonese Chicken Stock (page 256), hot

1 cup Hunts brand ketchup*

4 tablespoons light soy sauce

4 tablespoons Lee Kum Kee brand chili garlic sauce

4 tablespoons rice vinegar

4 tablespoons sugar

* Yes, this recipe has KETCHUP in it! And guess what? Ketchup is a VERY common ingredient in many Asian recipes. Not weird . . . not tastily weird at all.

Combine all ingredients in a mixing bowl (or 22-quart plastic Cambro containers, like we do) until it becomes one unified homogenous mixture of red chili sauce. It should taste spicy, sweet, and savory and not too ketchup-y.

BUTTERMILK BEER BEIGNETS

Developed specifically for our Singaporean Chili Crab dish, these beignets are savory pillows of donut deliciousness made specifically to sop up all sorts of sauces—the Malaysian Chicken Curry, the Braised and Caramelized Vietnamese Coco Pork Belly, and especially the Singaporean Chili Crab sauce—or ANY DISH with sauce! HOORAY!

2–4 SERVINGS

BALLS OUT
40–80 SERVINGS

5¼ quarts all-purpose flour

5¼ quarts cornstarch

14 tablespoons kosher salt

2⅓ tablespoons sugar

9⅓ tablespoons baking powder

3½ quarts buttermilk

10½ cups COLD Asian light beer

1½ cups all-purpose flour

1½ cups cornstarch

1 tablespoon kosher salt

½ teaspoon sugar

2 teaspoons baking powder

1 cup buttermilk *

¾ cup COLD Asian light beer

* Pour in the buttermilk and beat with minimal folding, then let it sit for at least an hour. The liquids will mix and react on their own, ensuring the fluffiest of savory beignets in the LAND! If it's not fully incorporated afterwards, fold a bit more until it's one uniform batter.

---

1. Combine flour, cornstarch, salt, sugar, and baking powder in a large mixing bowl. Mix well.
2. Pour in buttermilk, then pour in beer. Gently fold in with a baking spatula. DO NOT WHISK. A whisk will introduce too much air into the dough, which will make the beignets too tough.
3. The temperature of the batter is important! Refrigerate 30 minutes before frying. The beignet will come out more airy and less dense if the batter is, as Foreigner reminds us, "cold as ice."
4. When the beignets are ready to fry, bring a pot of oil up to 350°F over medium-high heat. Scoop up the dough with an ice cream scoop, drop in the pot of oil, and fry for about 4½–5 minutes, constantly turning until the dough is a light golden brown.
5. To sure the beignets are cooked through, stick them with a long skewer. The skewer should be clean when you remove it. If it's not, continue to fry.
6. Remove and shake off excess oil, then set aside.

BLACK PEPPER CRAB

Among most Singaporeans we've met (and we've met a lot of them since making Singaporean Chili Crab), this crab seems to be the resounding favorite, even if the Singaporean Chili Crab is more internationally well known.

Truth be told, though: Thi also loves this more than the Singaporean Chili Crab. Nonetheless, we've only made this for special events; we haven't offered it at a Starry Kitchen iteration . . . yet.

BALLS OUT
40–80 SERVINGS

20 fresh Dungeness crabs, or equally large and meaty crab

5 quarts tapioca starch (or cornstarch if tapioca starch isn't readily available)

6¼ cups unsalted butter*

2½ cups minced garlic

3¾ cups Tellicherry black peppercorns, coarsely ground†

1⅔ tablespoons ground white pepper

2½ teaspoons five-spice powder

1¼ cups oyster sauce

2½ cups Chinese cooking wine

2½ cups Superconcentrated Cantonese Chicken Stock (page 256)

2–4 SERVINGS

1 fresh Dungeness crabs, or equally large and meaty crab

1 cup tapioca starch (or cornstarch if tapioca starch isn't readily available)

3 tablespoons Tellicherry black peppercorns, coarsely ground†

5 tablespoons unsalted butter*

2 tablespoons minced garlic

¼ teaspoon ground white pepper

2 pinches five-spice powder

1 tablespoon oyster sauce

2 tablespoons Chinese cooking wine

2 tablespoons Superconcentrated Cantonese Chicken Stock (page 256)

* If you have the patience, unsalted BROWN butter is even better. You can make some from unsalted butter, and then this dish will be an unstoppable force in your culinary repertoire.

† Usually, we aren't picky about black pepper, but this recipe is designed specifically for Tellicherry black peppercorns. So promise to try your bestest to get these— pretty please?!?

1. Prepare the crab as you would in the Singaporean Chili Crab recipe, including frying all the crab parts.
2. In a wok/pan on low-medium heat, dry stir-fry the black peppercorn until fragrant. Remove from pan, and set aside.
3. Melt butter in wok/pan on low heat. Add garlic and sauté until brown. Then combine with stir-fried black pepper, white pepper, five-spice powder, oyster sauce, Chinese wine, and chicken stock.

4. Increase to high heat and toss in crab. Stir-fry until crab is hot to the touch and fully coated in all that flavorful peppery amazingness. Remove from heat, reconstruct in a bowl, and serve.

Oh yeah, get ready to be popular with every Singaporean person on your block . . . or move to a more predominant Singaporean neighborhood to make that happen!

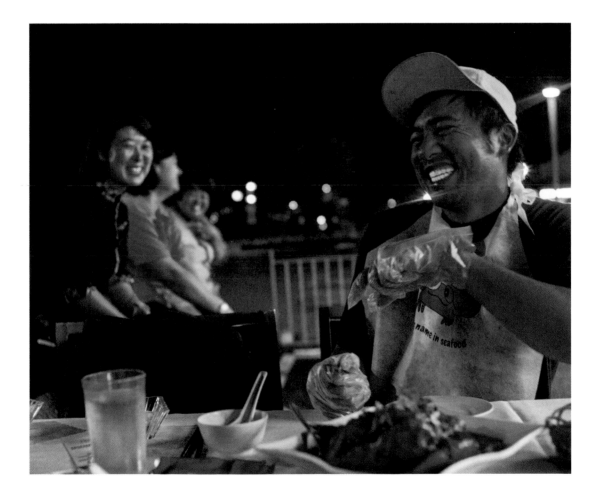

HOW TO EAT A CRAB

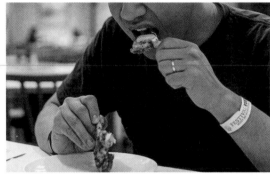

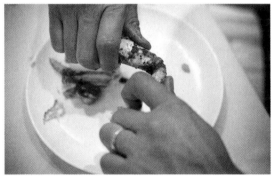

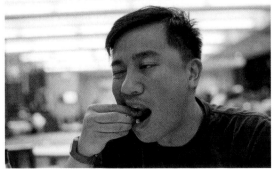

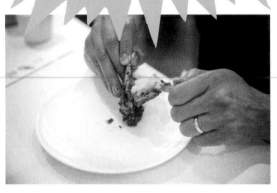

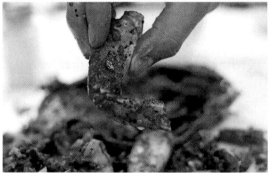

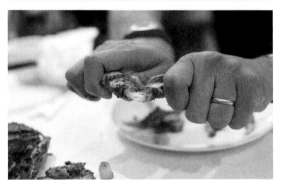

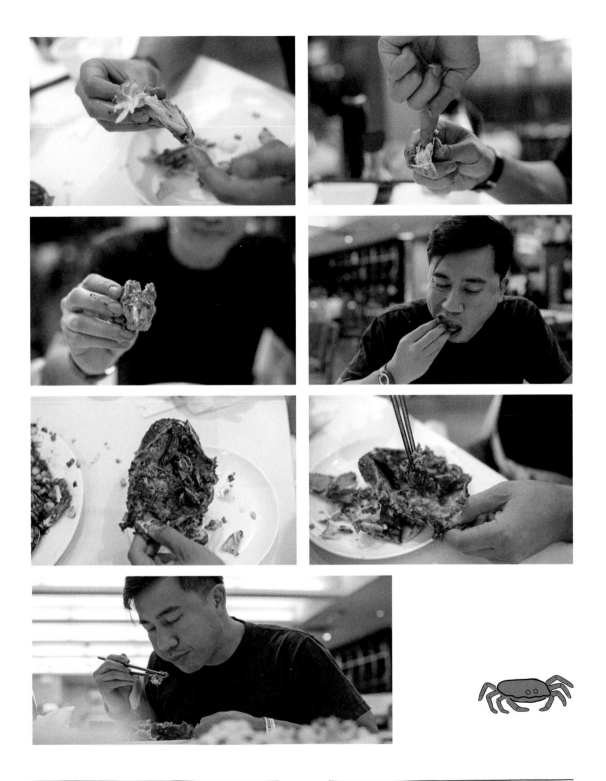

SECOND POP-UP / BUTTON MASH

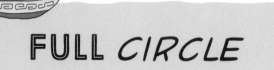

FULL *CIRCLE*

IN THE MIDDLE OF WRITING THIS BOOK, I GOT A CALL FROM GOLDEN VOICE, WHO RUNS THE COACHELLA VALLEY MUSIC AND ARTS FESTIVAL. COACHELLA BRINGS IN MORE THAN ONE HUNDRED THOUSAND PEOPLE PER DAY OVER THREE DAYS THROUGHOUT THE TWO WEEKENDS. IN RECENT YEARS, AS VIP TICKETS STARTED GOING FOR ABOUT $900 FOR THE WEEKEND, ORGANIZERS BEGAN PUSHING TO CATER TO THE MORE AFFLUENT AND HARD-CORE LA FOODIE. THIS MEANS THAT EVERY FOOD PLAYER IN LA, INCLUDING THE LIKES OF EGGSLUT, GUERRILLA TACOS, PHORAGE, BEER BELLY, RAMEN HOOD, AND MEXICALI TACO, HAS BEEN OR WILL BE INVITED TO TEST THEIR METTLE AT COACHELLA.

Coachella 2016 for us was one of the worst experiences I've ever had in the history of Starry Kitchen and in my life. I know I'll sound like an alcoholic who says he's not an alcoholic, but I can assure you, I'm not the kind of person who cracks and gets humbled easily. But Coachella did that to me in a blow so swift that just the thought of it still depresses me.

I mean, we planned for three months and spent almost $15k on rentals, deposits, equipment, hotels, and whatever else we needed before we got out there. I felt like a crack addict when we ran out of money and had to tap into the money we were saving for our newly born (and so fucking CUTE) baby boy Cillían. I promised myself and Thi that all would be fine and we would make it back. We made projections, we made plans, we had meetings upon meetings, we got a last-minute refrigerated truck rental with our friend Ilan Hall . . . we were good to go.

As much as I'm sure this is going to sound like dirty garbage (and the people who run these things ain't gonna like it), part of the problem is just how chaotic EVERYTHING is leading up to such events. Details and dates

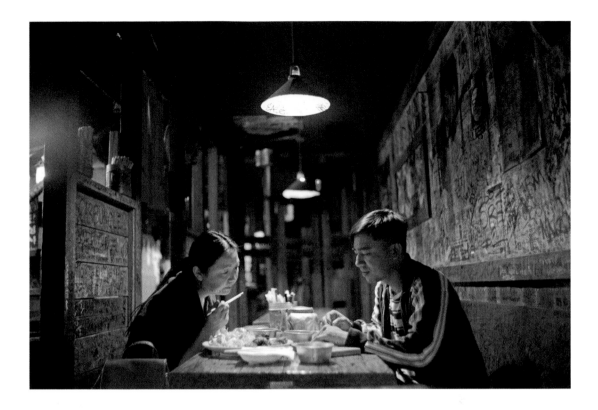

change so frequently that you're forced into a whirlwind of chaos that you can never control. But by that point, you're already in, so you can't do anything but play along.

A better way to put it: When running a business of any kind, part of your success is how much you can reduce the amount of unpredictability and the number of variables on the basis of your personal experience and the lessons you learned gaining that experience. The way to get ahead and succeed is to be able to anticipate and stay ahead of catastrophe.

Concerts: Instead of a six-sided die, you're tossing more like a twenty-sided one. Concerts force you out of reason and logic, and you can either go with the flow and just deal with it . . .

or crack. I promise you, I'm the kind of person who goes with the flow, but Coachella also ended up cracking me.

Moving your restaurant far away from home and creating a menu that's both appealing and executable is not an easy . . . fuck it, it's simply a fucking HARD feat to plan and execute. I mean, Starry Kitchen isn't hamburgers (even though we DO make a damn fine Classic Double Cheeseburger), hotdogs, chicken strips, funnel cakes, fried chicken, or anything with one or two words that concert kids can mentally take in in a highly suggestive state helped by admittedly fun recreational substances. It's not easy for any concertgoer to just walk up and get what he or she wants. And Crispy Tofu Balls, no matter how popular they are for us in the niche of the hard-core LA foodie community, hardly incite a manic reaction from people, like girls screaming and fainting at the sight of Michael Jackson back in the 1980s. Plus we're pan-Asian in influence, so I couldn't really agree to have a sign that just said "Chinese Food," "Orange Chicken," or "Chow Mein" in big letters (I would love to have a sign that says "Asian Food That White People Love More Than They Think They Would," but that's too many words . . . among other "things." Ha-ha.)

The same goes for our name. Yeah, foodie hipsters in LA might have heard of Starry Kitchen, but if these concert kids were even somewhat educated, that name might make them think of Van Gogh's *Starry Night* instead of food.

A rule: Real estate and location are EVERYTHING—even at a concert. You want to be near ALL the other food stands. People want options. They want to peruse what's available among the festival foods before the next performance of some EDM artist who sounds like the previous EDM artist, who has a ton of Instagram followers and can hit "Play" as easily as the previous DJ. "At a smaller concert we had worked, we were given what we thought was "prime real estate" as the sole food vendor next to the bar (the real star of any show). But we found out very quickly that people just wanted to get inebriated, and when they wanted to eat, they checked out the row of food outside the venue. They wouldn't come back to us!

I yearned to be there with the crowd, having the time of their lives. But there I was, Asian-squatting in the back of a refrigerated truck . . .

Funny thing: The same thing happened at Coachella for the first weekend. We were given the "prime real estate" as the sole vendor next to the coveted and HUGE craft beer bar. As arrogant as I am, I am very HAPPY to be proven wrong for the sake of success and business, so I was willing to roll the dice. Unfortunately, I hated being right in this case. It was a real struggle to get people to notice us and consider eating our food. And it wasn't for lack of trying. My team worked hard to get people's attention, and I made custom Starry Kitchen condoms to hand out. I don't like being that guy who complains while he's just sitting around waiting for someone to fix a problem. I ALWAYS think we can affect change.

But nothing changed until the first night of the first weekend of Coachella. I was on the other side of the concert grounds catching up with my colleagues in the LA food scene when I got a call from Monica, who works for me. She said, "Nguyen, you're not going to like this—you need to come back here."

What did that translate to? We had lost our golf cart because one of my guys broke a cardinal rule of golf carts (which he honestly didn't know), which is, you don't give anyone a ride in the trailer of the cart because people can fall off and get run over. My guy, no matter how earnestly he meant it, pissed off not just any security guard, but the head of ALL Coachella security when he caught him doing just that. Oh, and then I also found out that this golf cart event happened shortly after a woman had been killed by being run over by a commercial vehicle in the same back streets of Coachella on which our golf carts traveled, which effectively put all Coachella into golf cart security lockdown. This also meant that any infraction, no matter how small, was taken no less than incredibly seriously.

Thus our golf cart got confiscated, effective immediately for BOTH weekends of Coachella. Problem: ALL our product was in a refrigerated truck in a parking lot about a five-minute golf cart ride from our booth.

I scrambled to work my magic, but it was to no avail.

The next morning my staff started running back and forth with a flatbed dolly on the dusty desert roads. I could tell this was a bad idea and would wear and tear my staff like nothing else throughout the day. So I continued scrambling, talking to everyone who might have influence or could direct me to someone who could. Nothing.

My friends at Bling Bling Dumpling, however, ended up letting me borrow their cart, but only for a short time and about two hours after we really needed it. I was on a path to depression. I couldn't control any of it, and what little grasp I had left was getting looser, while the chasm between me and my normal amount of sanity grew exponentially. This was not good.

Even worse, our Crispy Tofu Balls—the thing that we're most well known for—were going bad. We had to dump most of them in a flash and start the process of making them all over again.

When I finally got that golf cart from Bling Bling, I already felt defeated. It was too little, too late. I was worn down. I couldn't hold a

smile to motivate my crew, who were being pushed harder than they should have been. This was the fucking shitter.

I finally made it to our refrigerated truck in what was the first trip back there without having to haul ass and run back and forth. It was already sundown. I opened up the truck. I found the tofu. I began cutting open tofu boxes to drain and press the tofu to make more balls. I could see the lights of Coachella in what seemed like a whole country away and listened to the crowd go crazy as Ice Cube performed. I yearned to be there with the crowd, having the time of their lives. But there I was, Asian-squatting in the back of a refrigerated truck, nearly on the verge of tears, being in a very lonely place and having the revelation that no matter how many times I've been written up in and reported by local, regional, and national press of all kinds, I and almost any restaurateur/chef could never escape the fact that when push comes to shove, we'll always be doing what it takes to feed the masses that get us that press and publicity no matter how big or small we are because THAT is our trade. In my case, it was just me, humbly Asian-squatting and cutting open tofu boxes while holding back tears because at the end of the day, what else could I do? Who else was going to do this?

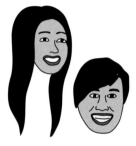

SINGAPOREAN CHILI CRAB GUMBO

You have NO idea how long I wanted to make this recipe a reality. Ever since I escaped Hurricane Gustav in 2008, I dreamed about making our version of a Deep South Cajun-approved stick-to-your-ribs gumbo. The deep-flavor chocolatey Dark Roux is the basis for this incredibly complex gumbo that uses the same sauce as the Singaporean Chili Crab but is married to lots of homey Asian herbs and spices and everything nice(s).

2–4 SERVINGS

½ cup ½ inch diced mountain yams (aka *nagaimo*)

1 cup diced yellow onions

½ cup finely chopped Chinese celery stalk*

1 tablespoon chopped garlic

½ pound andouille sausage

¾ cup Dark Roux (page 241)

4 cups Superconcentrated Cantonese Chicken Stock (page 256)

1½ whole bay leaves

½ tablespoon Worcestershire sauce

2 pinches of cayenne pepper

¾ teaspoon kosher salt

⅓ teaspoon fresh ground pepper

½ pound crab meat

2 cups Chili Crab Sauce (page 212)

¼ cup chopped scallions

1 tablespoon fresh thyme leaves

½ tablespoon chopped Thai basil

1 tablespoon gumbo filé powder (aka sassafras)

½ cup ¼-inch diced freshwater chestnuts or jicama (optional)†

½ tablespoon chicken bouillon

* Chinese celery is much smaller than traditional celery and tastes different, too. Oh, and cut off and do something else with them . . . but not in this dish! ☺

† If you grew up eating only Americanized Chinese food, you most likely only had dried or not-so-freshwater chestnuts. If you can find and afford fresh water chestnuts, HOLY CRAP, you're in for a treat that I only recently discovered myself.

BALLS OUT
40–80 SERVINGS

4 quarts ½ inch diced mountain yams (aka *nagaimo*)

8 quarts diced yellow onions

4 quarts finely chopped Chinese celery stalk*

2 cups chopped garlic

16 pounds andouille sausage

6 quarts Dark Roux (page 241)

32 quarts Superconcentrated Cantonese Chicken Stock (page 256)

48 whole bay leaves

1 cup Worcestershire sauce

4 teaspoons cayenne pepper

½ cup kosher salt

¼ cup fresh ground pepper

16 pounds crab meat

16 quarts Chili Crab Sauce (page 212)

2 quarts chopped scallions

2 cups fresh thyme leaves

1 cup chopped Thai basil

2 cups gumbo filé powder (aka sassafras)

4 quarts ¼-inch diced freshwater chestnuts or jicama †

1 cup chicken bouillon

1. Bring a pot of water to a rolling boil over high heat. Prepare an ice water bath in a bowl while waiting for the water to boil. Parboil mountain yams for 1 minute. Remove, strain, and shock in ice water bath, while gently scrubbing the yams with your hands to get rid of the sliminess and starchiness. Drain and set aside.

2. Sauté diced onions, celery, and garlic in a pan until lightly brown. Set aside in another bowl.

3. Cut sausage into ¾-inch slices, then sauté until cooked through and lightly brown. Set aside in a different bowl.

4. In a stock pot, heat Dark Roux over medium-high heat, stirring constantly. Once the roux is hot, combine with sautéed onions, celery, and garlic. Next, slowly pour in chicken stock, whisking constantly to prevent lumps.

5. Add sautéed sausages, bay leaves, Worcestershire sauce, cayenne pepper, salt, and pepper.

6. If using canned crab, drain the liquid. Mix crab meat with the Chili Crab Sauce in yet another bowl, then combine the chili crab meat sauce along with scallions, thyme, and basil in the pot. Sprinkle in filé powder and mix thoroughly. Bring to a boil over high heat, stirring often, then decrease to a simmer once it boils. To reduce the gumbo to a desired rib-sticking thickness, adjust to medium heat, uncovered. Once reduced (to your pleasure), add yams, chestnuts, and chicken bouillon.

    Heat and mix before serving in a bowl . . . over rice . . . or in a red Solo cup with a big fat straw. Enjoy it, however you want!

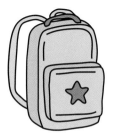

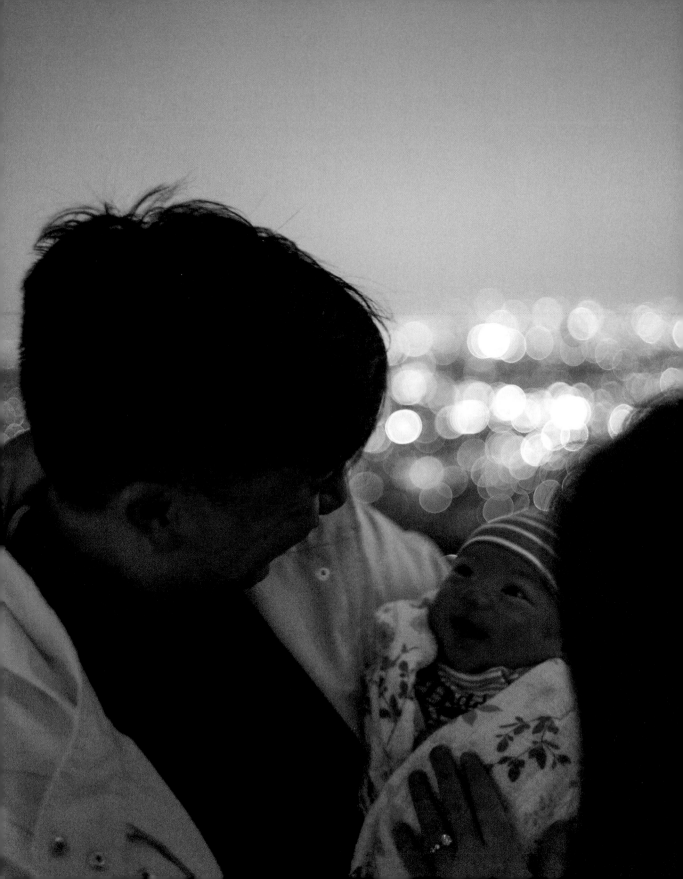

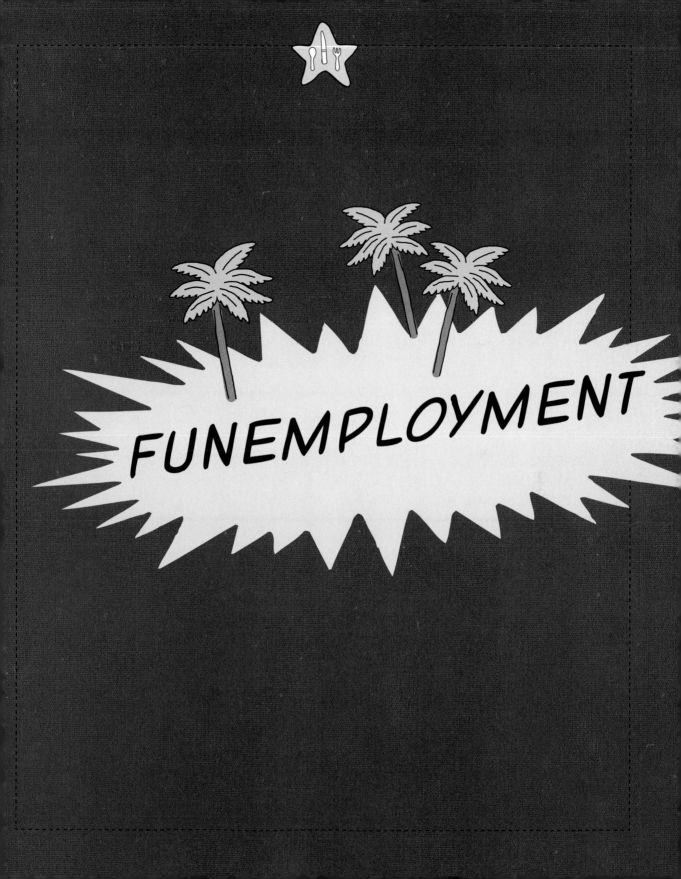

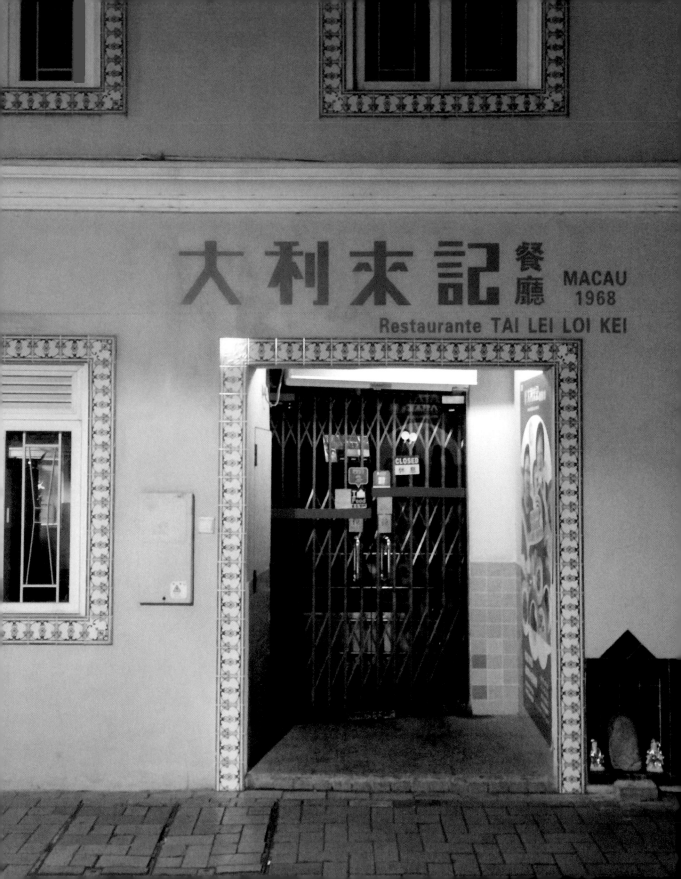

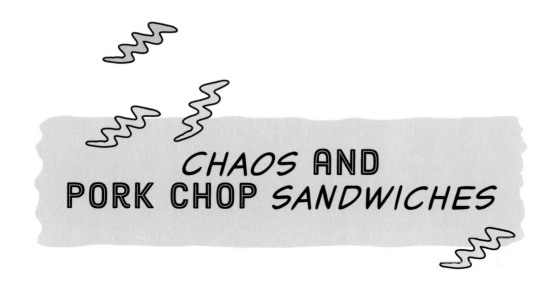

CHAOS AND PORK CHOP SANDWICHES

BEFORE I STARTED WRITING THIS BOOK, I PITCHED TO MY PUBLISHER THE IDEA OF VISITING ASIA WITH A PHOTOGRAPHER TO TAKE SCENIC SHOTS OF ASIAN COUNTRIES, ASIAN FOOD, AND—BECAUSE THE PHOTOGRAPHER WAS A FRIEND OF MINE—JUST GO BONKERS THROUGHOUT ASIA, ALL IN SERVICE OF THE BOOK.

Part of that plan was something I've obsessed about for almost a decade: the Tai Lei Loi Kei Macanese pork chop sandwich. This pork chop sandwich is pretty simple, but what's not so simple is the sandwich's backstory, or the rules of the place that sells it. Since I first heard about both, I have been fascinated with them and carried the regret of not trying this legendary sammie almost a decade ago.

The island country of Macau, a former Portuguese colony that is now under the control of the People's Republic of China, is famous for its fusion of Chinese and Portuguese culture, including the famous Portuguese egg tart (aka *natas* aka *po tat*), some of the most lavish

casinos, and an unabashed celebration of high-stakes gambling and high-end shopping. But all I cared about on my visit to the Macanese island of Taipa was the little stand that produced 300 bone-in pork chop sandwiches served on a sweet roll. People lined up all morning for this sandwich, and if you were number 301, you were out of luck, no two ways about it.

After first hearing about the Tai Lei Loi Kei pork chop stand in 2005, I KNEW I had to visit Taipa to try the sandwich. But, did I go right away? NOPE, because I wasn't as annoying as I am now. That is, not yet annoying enough to persuade Thi when we were in Hong Kong to wake up early enough to take a ferry over to Macau and hop in a cab for the drive to Taipa, just to wait in a line for the outside shot of getting two of these coveted pork chop sandwiches. Serves me right for being considerate.

Thi and I went to Hong Kong in late 2007 to announce our engagement and attend the weddings of two cousins. No time for Macau. Early the next year, I returned to Hong Kong on business, which didn't leave me any time to visit Macau. We started Starry Kitchen in 2009, which meant the poorhouse for many more years than most restaurateurs should have to endure. But through all this, I still couldn't stop thinking about that sandwich.

So when I persuaded my publisher that I had to go to Asia, I made sure to leave enough time to squeeze in an overnight trip to Macau to finally eat that motherfucking pork chop sandwich.

But to understand me is to understand that I'm overzealous and unreasonably ambitious beyond any logic or reason. (One can dream, right?!) I scheduled nine countries in fewer than three weeks. Though Macau was a focus of the trip, I could make it work only if I first visited three countries in two days—without sleeping. I flew sixteen hours to Shanghai for a seven-hour layover so I could be drenched in the downpour of China just to see the futuristic neon lights of the city. Then I took a two-hour flight to Singapore for another layover, this time a ten-hour one, just so I could hit some hawker stands in the muggy heat of Southeast Asia to comfort my craving for powerful and mouthwatering flavors. After getting drenched and sweating through my T-shirt, I devolved into a stinky walking cesspool (it was so bad that a flight attendant on the plane actually

took an aerosol can of air freshener and sprayed down the cabin five rows behind me and directly onto my feet) and THEN I drearily, finally flew into the island city of Taipa two days after leaving the States.

Waiting for my bus outside the Macau airport, I realized I needed to get going or I was going to drop. I figured it was time to take a cheap taxi two miles down the road. That seemed like the smartest, uncheapest decision I had made in a while. But none of the cab drivers knew how to find my Airbnb rental. Even though addresses were written in Portuguese, the cabbies only knew the Cantonese names. Since the extent of my Cantonese was "This tastes good" and "I don't speak Cantonese," directing cabbies around Taipa wasn't going to happen. Finally I found a cabbie who tolerated my lack of Cantonese enough to take me where I needed to go. So things were at last looking up. HUZZAH!

Now, before I continue I should mention that being a road warrior is not foreign to me. I LOVE the chaos and excitement of travel.

That said, one of my biggest pet peeves about traveling is cabbies trying to rip me off. And this cabbie hit my button immediately. I'm still mad at that guy! When we reached my destination, he started cursing me in Cantonese. And then I started yelling at him in English and my limited Cantonese, telling him how much I was going to pay him regardless of how much he wanted to charge me. As I was yelling at him, I could feel him letting his foot off of the brake. He was about to peel out and take me god-knows-where. I grabbed my bags, and as quickly as I got out of the cab, a lady jumped in, and the cabbie was already on his

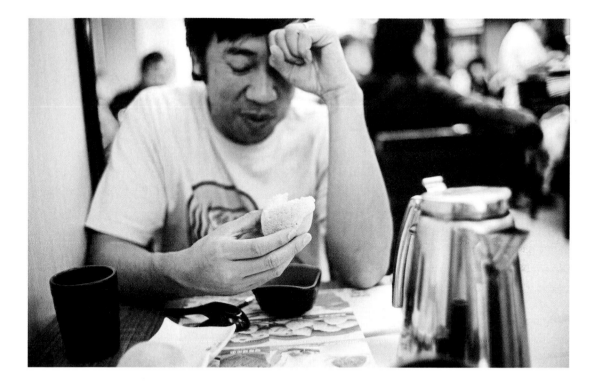

way. That's when I realized that I had left one of my phones in the back of the cab—the one with all the information I needed for the rest of my trip.

I was so mad! I was so livid! I was so screwed. I tried the public phones in the hotel near my Airbnb, but they were all disconnected. Fortunately, the hotel managers were incredibly gracious, especially considering that I wasn't even staying there. They got me a glass of water, set me up on their Wi-Fi, and left me alone as I tried every app known in the iCloud to track down, beep, whatever I could to get my phone back. I couldn't believe it. This was the first true night of my trip, and it couldn't have started off worse. I was exhausted, probably stranded, and at a total loss.

But, as I slowly started to calm down, a simple realization hit me: I thrive in chaos. This is what I had forgotten about myself. And this is what I realize about myself now. This is how Starry Kitchen survived through all the turmoil. This is one of the few intangible skills that is hard as hell to articulate but easy as anything for me to put into action: functioning in chaos. Against ALL odds and especially when I'm fucked, I get shit done. I don't cave in; I don't wallow; and I simply don't give a fuck about what normal logic tells me I can't make happen.

This idea was always in front of me and I finally grabbed it and finally owned it. This is who I am. It permeates my soul. Sitting there without my phone and facing the chaos before me, I became one . . . with me.

I went to my Airbnb, restored all my backed-up info to my other phone, which I use primarily for pictures, and then set out on foot to find my pork chop sandwich.

With my broken Cantonese, I searched for two long hours and asked a few local police officers about the highly elusive *chi pa bao*. At first they dismissed me, but of course through my sheer persistence (aka I just stared at them stupidly and mimicked eating a pork chop sandwich), they figured out what I wanted and pointed out the place four doors away.

Tai Lei Loi Kei has become so legendary that the business has expanded throughout Macau, Singapore, and other Asian regions. The flagship, while still near its original spot, has expanded into a beautifully yellow building that accommodates hungry customers all day. So much for having to be one of the lucky 300. But I didn't care. My trip wasn't just about that. I walked over, took selfies in front of the place, knowing full well that all this chaos and turmoil would be worth it if it opened in a few hours before I left the country. I returned to my Airbnb to sleep for three hours before I satisfied my unconditional love for a pork chop sandwich with an open bun and a juicy chop ready for my consumption and a mouthful of lovin'.

I woke up, packed up so that I was ready to leave just in case I came back very late from my sandwich excursion, and set off for my pork chop sammie of a lifetime. I got there at 7:30 A.M. No one was there yet. Five minutes later, this sweet old lady walked in, and like a crazy stalker I slipped in behind her and interrogated her with my broken Cantonese about when the place would open. 8:00 A.M.!

So I sat in front of the building. Watched the bread get delivered. Watched kids go to school. Watched buses take locals to work. Avoided a street cleaner and marveled about traversing an ocean, using two different phones, trekking through three countries for THIS sandwich—an adventure never to be replicated by anyone else again, including me.

When 8 A.M. finally rolled around, I casually walked in and sat down like I was a local there for my daily coffee, soccer match, and pork chop sandwich. I ordered two—one to savor and make love to with my mouth right then and there, and one to take with me on the road. Then I heard a microwave turn on. But it simply didn't matter anymore. I was there! Five minutes later, they were in my hands. That first bite of a moist sweet roll paired with tender pork marinated in five-spice and other seasoning overcame my tired soul and rejuvenated me . . . and then I knew that the next three weeks were going to be full of chaotic greatness.

I scarfed that pork chop sandwich down. Devoured it. Mouth-gasmed to it to the *n*th degree. I was more than happy. I was on a different plane of enlightenment, not only because it was delicious and entirely worth the effort, but also because I never gave up on it, not once after ten years of obsessing over it, and when I finally got to taste it, I also got to celebrate and acknowledge in full the chaotic order I live in with Starry Kitchen—all of its crazy successes and even crazier adventures. Everything flooded through my mouth into my being.

All that from a Macanese pork chop sandwich . . .

BRAISED PORK BELLY WITH VIETNAMESE FERMENTED SHRIMP PASTE AND LEMONGRASS

This dish is SO deliciously funky. This might be funkier than the Ribeye Satay Noodles, and I love both, so I don't mind that at all.

2–4 SERVINGS

BALLS OUT
40–80 SERVINGS

3¾ cups fermented shrimp paste

3¾ cups sugar

3⅓ tablespoons crushed red pepper flakes

20 pounds pork belly, diced into 1-inch cubes

6 cups plus 3 tablespoons minced lemongrass

1¼ cups minced garlic

3 tablespoons fermented shrimp paste	½ teaspoon crushed red pepper flakes	5 tablespoons minced lemongrass
3 tablespoons sugar	1 pound pork belly, diced into 1-inch cubes	1 tablespoon minced garlic

1. Combine shrimp paste, sugar, and red pepper flakes in a bowl and mix well.
2. In a pan/wok, sauté pork belly without any additional oil on medium heat for 5–7 minutes. Once the fat from the pork starts to render, add lemongrass and garlic. Stir-fry until garlic and lemongrass turn golden brown.
3. Now add shrimp paste mixture. Stir well, reduce to medium-low heat, and simmer for 10 minutes, or until sauce thickens.

Remove from heat, eat with rice, and get ready to bring in da FUNK!

JAPANESE CURRY ROUX

I call Japanese curry the "gateway curry."

When my uncle Frankie first took me to a Curry House restaurant in Southern California (when I was still living in the Great State of Texas, Y'ALL!), I immediately fell in love with Japanese curry. I fell even deeper in love through our sheer curry determination when we finally made our own!

Japanese curry is tempered with honey, apples, and all sorts of nice and sweet things, which makes it less pungent and more palatable than other more extreme curries.

BALLS OUT
40–80 SERVINGS

6 cups plus 2 tablespoons Dark Roux (page 241)

1¼ cups Indian curry powder

1¼ cups garam masala

6⅔ tablespoons smoked paprika

1¼ cups Worcestershire sauce

1¼ cups tomato sauce

FOR CURRY SAUCE:

7½ quarts water

½ teaspoon scorpion pepper sauce (optional . . . VERY optional)

2–4 SERVINGS

5 tablespoons Dark Roux (page 241)

1 tablespoon Indian curry powder

1 tablespoon garam masala

1 teaspoon smoked paprika

1 tablespoon Worcestershire sauce

1 tablespoon tomato sauce

FOR CURRY SAUCE:

1½ cups water

1 dash scorpion pepper sauce (optional . . . VERY optional)

1. Heat up Dark Roux in a pot over low-medium heat to loosen it up a bit. Then add curry powder, garam masala, and paprika. Mix evenly. Then add Worcestershire sauce and tomato sauce until completely and fully incorporated. Remove from heat. The final product will have a similar texture and feel as the cold Dark Roux, just with Japanese curry flavor. Set aside or chill in fridge until you get the hankerin' for some deliciously hearty CURRY!

2. When you DO get that hankerin', combine the finished Japanese Curry Roux and water in a pot over medium heat. Stir until a smooth consistency. Comforting curry at its very finest.

3. We love to add some heat with scorpion pepper sauce, which Davan Maharaj from the *LA Times* introduced me to. (Don't worry, he's the only kind of fancy friend we have; we don't know anyone else "cool" LOL.)

4. Don't be deceived if the curry looks a little thin with whatever you choose to stew/cook it with. The minute you remove from heat, the curry thickens up in quite a lovely way.

I love this curry so much that just writing about it makes me feel euphoric . . . *Ahhhhhhhhh!*

CHICKEN FRIED STEAK [AKA COUNTRY FRIED STEAK]

There's nothing Asian about this classic down-home and as-Southern-as-it-gets dish—until you top it with Japanese Curry Roux. Then it's a whole different Asian ballgame!

2–4 SERVINGS

BALLS OUT
40–80 SERVINGS

80 cube steaks*

5 quarts self-rising flour†

1⅔ cups garlic powder

1⅔ cups onion powder

1⅔ cups chicken bouillon

13⅓ tablespoons cracked black pepper

6⅔ tablespoons cayenne pepper (optional)

1⅔ cups kosher salt

60 large eggs

10 cups buttermilk

---

4 cube steaks*

2 cups self-rising flour†

4 teaspoons garlic powder

4 teaspoons onion powder

4 teaspoons chicken bouillon

2 teaspoons cracked black pepper

1 teaspoon cayenne pepper (optional, for a lil HEEEEEEEEEEEEEAT!)

4 teaspoons kosher salt

3 large eggs

½ cup buttermilk

* This is typically a cheap cut of top-round steak that is machine processed, tenderized, and flattened out, but if you can't find it you can get any steak, like a nice ribeye, and pound the crap out of it . . . even though a ribeye is deserving of your wholesome unadulterated consumption too.

† If you ain't got self-rising, you can MAKE it; just mix 2 cups flour, 1 teaspoon kosher salt, and 3 teaspoons baking powder—and you gots it!

---

1. Even if your beef has already been machine pounded, you'll still want to pound (the crap out of) it with a meat tenderizer until it's flattened even more, still firm, but not completely limp. After pounding, beef should be almost double in surface area and size, and about ½-inch thick or a little less.

2. From here on out, make sure all your bowls are large enough to dredge the flattened-out steaks.

3. Next, add self-rising flour to a bowl and season with garlic powder, onion powder, chicken bouillon, black pepper, cayenne pepper, and kosher salt. Taste the seasoned flour—THIS is how your Chicken Fried Steak is going to taste. Feel free to season more to taste, but don't forget that you might eat this with some sauce, like gravy or Japanese Curry Roux, so don't make it TOO flavorful and salty.

4. Beat eggs in another bowl and mix with buttermilk.

5. Now for some messy double-dredging fun. Take a steak and fully coat in flour bowl, shake off excess, dip into buttermilk egg wash, then dip it BACK into flour. That's the pro move, y'all!

6. Heat up a pan/skillet with 1 inch oil on medium-high heat to 350°F.

7. Be careful not to heat the oil too high or it's gonna burn the batter. And no one (except a select few I can't speak for) wants to eat super-burnt Chicken Fried Steak! Oh, I know there are some steak purists out there, but in this case, please just accept the fact that this isn't a normal steak and it's gonna be well done . . . and that's that!

8. Once the oil is ready, drop one of your nicely double-dredged steaks into your pan. Fry 3–4 minutes, or until red meat juice starts to bubble out of the top of the steak. The steak should have a nice golden brown coating underneath. Next, gently turn over steak with a long fork, tongs, or long wooden chopsticks (like I do). Cook another 3–4 minutes or until fully golden brown, then remove from pan, shake off excess oil, and drip dry on a paper towel–lined plate or an elevated grate over a lined baking sheet.

9. Repeat for remaining cutlets.

10. While frying the other steaks, keep the cooked steaks warm in the oven at 170°F, but only if you have a grate and pan to keep them elevated. If they sit on a flat pan in the oven, the steaks will swim in their own oils and then they'll have a soggy underbelly, making you question why you fried them in the first place. Why? WHY?!?!?

And now you can enjoy steak as it's sometimes meant to be eaten—fried like an extra-tasty piece of crispy chicken. Eat as is or serve with various gravy recipes you can find online (I love peppery turkey neck gravy myself, if anyone's asking), but my real favorite way to enjoy it is with a Japanese Curry Roux and side of rice! I'm going to (will the idea into reality and) open that cart one day—just you watch!

Banh mi, o' banh mi! One of the most beloved culinary gifts my country has bestowed on the world, and another example of French colonialism at its finest, though our version leaves out the traditional Gallic-inspired ingredients of paté, French (Buerdell brand) butter, and very often delicious headcheese, which isn't even cheese . . . enjoy!

2–4 SERVINGS

BALLS OUT
40–80 SERVINGS

**GINGER
GARLIC AIOLI:**

1¼ cups Starry Kitchen Mayo (page 254)

1⅔ tablespoons finely minced ginger

3⅓ tablespoons finely minced garlic

1⅔ tablespoons sugar

1¼ teaspoons kosher salt

1⅔ tablespoons lime juice

THE SAMMIE:

20 loaves French-Vietnamese bread or Mexican bolillos

10 cups medium shredded cabbage*

Pickled Shredded Carrots and Daikon (page 250)

40 sprigs cilanto

10 jalapenos, thinly sliced on a bias

**GINGER
GARLIC AIOLI:**

5 tablespoons Starry Kitchen Mayo (page 254)

¼ teaspoon finely minced ginger

½ teaspoon finely minced garlic

¼ teaspoon sugar

Pinch of kosher salt

¼ teaspoon lime juice

THE SAMMIE:

1 loaf French-Vietnamese bread or Mexican bolillos

½ cup medium shredded cabbage*

Pickled Shredded Carrots and Daikon (page 250)

2 sprigs cilanto

½ jalapeño, thinly sliced on a bias

Sriracha sauce (optional)

* Not even close to a traditional filling for a banh mi, but we like to include it in ours for texture and a little more filling

1. Mix all ginger garlic aioli ingredients in a bowl. Set aside in a container that can be refrigerated.
2. Slice open bread from one end to the other, but only enough to open it up and stuff great ingredients in. Spread bread with aioli. Stuff with cabbage, cilantro, Pickled Shredded Carrots and Daikon, and jalapeño slices. Stick whatever meat or protein source you want in there. Then, if you want (I know I do), add some sriracha across and go to town.

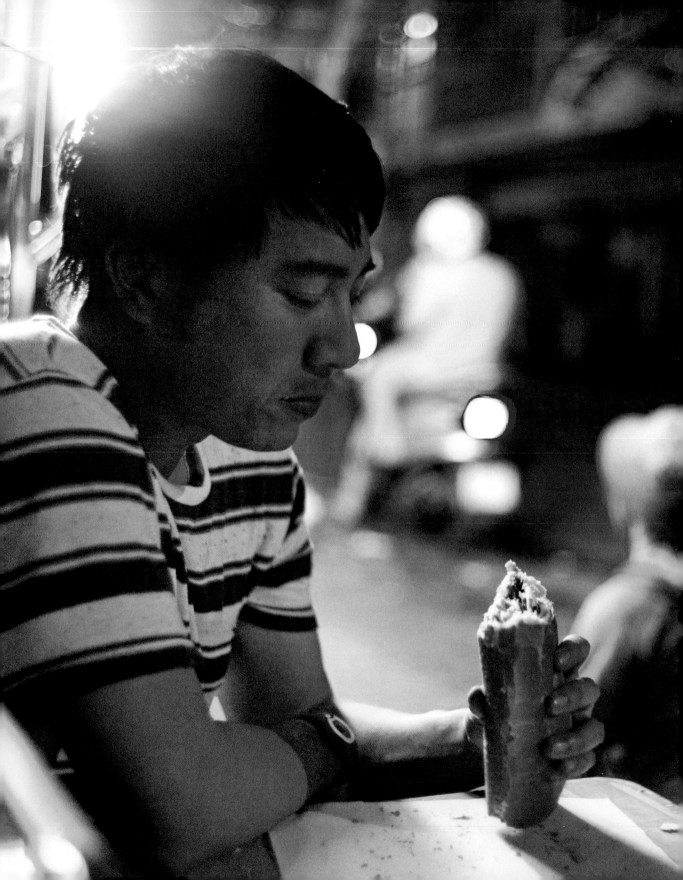

BEEF TALLOW / RENDERED BEEF FAT

Extra-tasty fat—it makes food and America better. It will also help you cut back on purchasing vegetable/canola/corn/patchouli/hipster oils, while also making every dish you cook using a deeper, more delicious, and super-less-vegetarian tasty beef fat.

Trimmed beef fat—as much as you can spare from a ribeye or any other beef or beef dish

Throw as much fat as you can into a pot or pan, and over a low to medium-low heat, let it BUUUUUUUUUUUUUUUUUURN!

Well, not really. Don't fill the kitchen with smoke! Once the fat darkens from white to a deep brown, discard the solid fat and save the liquid fat for the unknown future flavor awaiting you.

I am literally the biggest fuckup I KNOW!

—INTRODUCTION

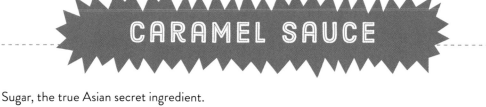

CARAMEL SAUCE

Sugar, the true Asian secret ingredient.

BALLS OUT
40–80 SERVINGS

5 quarts sugar

5 cups plus 10 cups water

2–4 SERVINGS

1 cup sugar   ¼ cup plus ½ cup water

1. Heat sugar and ¼ cup water in a saucepan over medium-low heat for 12–15 minutes. Let sugar melt. Do not stir. It will sizzle, so be careful around it.
2. While waiting, set up a large bowl or sink with enough hot water to dip the bottom of the pan into it.
3. Once mixture caramelizes into a dark black color and turns super-thick like molasses, dip the bottom of the pan in the hot water bath to stop the cooking process. Be careful of water spilling into the pan and watch out for the steam as well.
4. Add remaining water to pan. Be careful. It will also sizzle. *Yikes!*
5. Next, remove pan from water bath. Bring pan back to your stove over medium heat, stirring until the caramel dissolves in water. The flavor should be bittersweet.

   Use this sauce for the delicious recipes that call for it, such as Braised and Caramelized Vietnamese Coco Pork Belly, and Bun Cha Hanoi.

COCO RICO
VIETNAMESE FISH SAUCE

I am Vietnamese, I like fish sauce . . . BUT Vietnamese fish sauce is NOT just plain fish sauce. It's far more complex—a delicate balance between water, fish sauce, sugar, and the right amount of acidity. And (every Vietnamese person including me thinks) it's AH-MAAAAAAAAAZING with everything!

BALLS OUT
40–80 SERVINGS

5¼ quarts sugar

5¼ quarts fish sauce

4¼ cups minced garlic

67 Thai chilies, stemmed and finely chopped

7 quarts Coco Rico brand soda

7 quarts key lime or lime juice

2–4 SERVINGS

¾ cup sugar

¾ cup fish sauce

2½ tablespoons minced garlic

2 Thai chilies, stemmed and finely chopped

1 cup Coco Rico brand soda

1 cup key lime or lime juice

1. In a pot, dissolve sugar into fish sauce on low heat. Remove from heat and add garlic, chilies, soda, and key lime juice. Stir it all in, taste it (it should be lightly sweet and barely fishlike savory, with a little bit of tanginess), and adjust to your liking; but remember, the main ingredients are sugar, water, and acid/limes. If you have too much of one ingredient, you will have to balance the flavor by adding appropriate amounts of the other two main ingredients.

2. Let it sit for 30 minutes before using.

   Refrigerate unused sauce and serve with anything and everything—it will get better, spicier, and more Vietnamese-approved over time.

DARK ROUX

Though there are different stages of a roux, we prefer a dark chocolate roux, which is deeper in flavor (and color and consistency) and nuttier in aroma. When you smell the Starry Kitchen-approved roux in your kitchen, you'll understand the difference and will thank us later.

Ⓐ Ⓐ Ⓐ

The yield varies, depending on the kind of oil. We most often use cottonseed oil, but when we want to splurge (it's more expensive), butter is always deeper in flavor. Oh man, I gotta sit down just thinking about how much better it is with butter!—it's THAT much better.

BALLS OUT
40–80 SERVINGS

12½ quarts all-purpose flour

7½ quarts cooking oil or melted butter

2–4 SERVINGS

2½ cups all-purpose flour	1½ cups cooking oil or melted butter

1. Get ready to test your forearm endurance. There's no quitting once you start, but if you aren't able to stick with it all the way through, OK, you CAN remove the pot/pan off the heat when you need a break. When you're ready to stir again, return the roux to the heat. No matter how many breaks you take, though, it still requires the same amount of total time and energy.

2. Pour flour into saucepan or pot with deep sides over medium heat. Mix with a whisk or wooden spoon, constantly stirring to ensure flour doesn't sit for too long in any one spot. If the flour sits, it will burn, which will ruin the roux.

3. Continue to stir for 10 minutes, or until flour turns a golden brown. Introduce oil in a constant stream, while stirring. It will start out "blonde," and start to slowly get darker over time. Once the roux turns a shade of and exhibits the consistency of chocolate (which could be 20 minutes to an hour depending on how much flour you're working with), stop stirring and remove from heat. It will continue to darken as it cools. You'll see the color and the thickness magically change right before your eyes.

   Continue to let cool, then transfer into a container for immediate or later use and store.

GINGER SESAME SAKE SAUCE

I still remember making this at our old illegal+underground apartment back in the "good ol' days." This is great with salads, and as a marinade, but really it was made for the Lemongrass Tofu (page 14).

BALLS OUT
40–80 SERVINGS

1¼ cups sugar

5 cups rice vinegar

7 cups plus 2 tablespoons cooking oil

2½ cups sesame oil

2½ cups light soy sauce

2½ cups sake

5 cups grated or finely minced ginger

2–4 SERVINGS

2 tablespoons sugar

½ cup rice vinegar

⅞ cup plus 1 tablespoon cooking oil

¼ cup sesame oil

¼ cup light soy sauce

¼ cup sake

½ cup grated or finely minced ginger

Dissolve sugar in rice vinegar over low heat. Once it's dissolved, remove from heat and add vegetable oil, sesame oil, soy sauce, sake, and ginger and stir.

And yeah, that's it. Dig in . . . however you want to use, toss, top, or eat it like our Director of Operations, Monica, who loves to eat it with plain old rice!

HONEY BOURBON CREAM SAUCE

This is liquid crack of the gods . . . that is all. (mic drop)

2–4 SERVINGS

BALLS OUT
40–80 SERVINGS

½ cup cornstarch

1 cup plus 7 cups heavy whipping cream

3 cups sugar

1 cup honey bourbon whiskey*

4 tablespoons real vanilla extract

1 tablespoon cornstarch

2 tablespoons plus 14 tablespoons heavy whipping cream

6 tablespoons sugar

2 tablespoons honey bourbon whiskey*

½ tablespoon real vanilla extract

* A certain brand that rhymes with "Smack Saniels" works, if you want a suggestion

1. In a small bowl, mix cornstarch and 2 tablespoons cream into a slurry. Set aside.

2. Heat sugar, bourbon, and the remaining cream in a pan over medium heat to dissolve sugar and burn off the alcohol. Once sugar is dissolved and alcohol has burned off (bubbling will be at a minimum), add slurry. Stir until the cream thickens. To get rid of lumps, strain through a chinois or fine-mesh strainer.

   Let it cool, use as a dip (like for the Five-Spice Apple Fritters), then store for the next dessert rager.

PICKLING LIQUID

We like pickles. We like to pickle. We like sweeter pickles. And we like (most of) you.☺ (As long as you don't fuck with our recipes too much.) But really, that's how we started all our shenanigans—by doing it *our* way, fucking around—and you should TOO, so PLEASE fuck with our recipes, and then let us know what you do. We wanna try it too!

BALLS OUT
40–80 SERVINGS

4 quarts cold water

5 quarts sugar

2 cups kosher salt

5 quarts distilled white vinegar

2–4 SERVINGS

1 cup cold water

1¼ cups sugar

2 tablespoons kosher salt

1¼ cups distilled white vinegar

In a pot, combine water, sugar, and salt over medium heat. Stir until sugar dissolves. Be careful not to boil. Remove from heat, add vinegar, and get ready to be the pickling prince or princess of your block, "Your Majesty!"

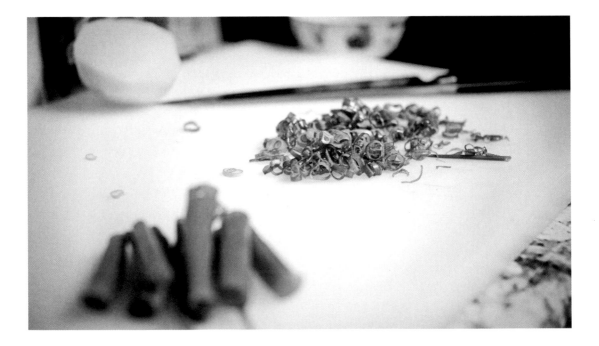

ESCABECHE

These pickled jalapeños (and carrots and onions and sometimes cauliflower) are one of the best pick-led condiments you can get at the many authentic taco stands (at all hours of the day or night) in the great city of Los Angeles . . . and one of the great gifts we got from our original Oaxacan staff.

BALLS OUT
40–80 SERVINGS

8 quarts sliced jalapeños

4 quarts sliced carrots

3 quarts sliced yellow or white onions

2 cups bay leaves (loosely packed)

1 cup kosher salt

¼ cup black peppercorns

2 tablespoons oregano

2 tablespoons cumin powder

2 tablespoons whole cloves

2 cups whole garlic cloves

2 cups thinly sliced garlic

1 tablespoon coriander seeds

20 star anise pods

16 quarts Pickling Liquid (page 244)

2–4 SERVINGS

1 cup sliced jalapeños

½ cup sliced carrots

⅓ cup sliced yellow or white onions

2 whole bay leaves

1½ teaspoons kosher salt

⅓ teaspoon black peppercorns

3 pinches oregano

3 pinches cumin powder

3 pinches whole cloves

3 whole garlic cloves

3 teaspoons thinly sliced garlic

1 pinch coriander seeds

1 star anise pod

3 cups Pickling Liquid (page 244)

1. Combine everything but Pickling Liquid in a container that can handle boiling hot liquids.

2. Bring Pickling Liquid to a full boil in a pot over high heat. Remove from heat and immediately pour over ingredients. Cover with plastic wrap. Make sure the wrap is flush across and pushed down onto the liquid surface so the veggies are completely submerged. Let cool to room temperature before refrigerating.

PICKLED KOHLRABI

A vegetable that looks like my bedhead from the '90s, but far tastier (I'm sure most would agree).

BALLS OUT
40–80 SERVINGS

5 pounds kohlrabi

Kosher salt, for cleaning

10 quarts Pickling Liquid (page 244)

2–4 SERVINGS

| ½ pound kohlrabi | Kosher salt, for cleaning | 4 cups Pickling Liquid (page 244) |

1. Cut leaves and stems off kohlrabi and wash them and kohlrabi well to get rid of any dirt or sand. Discard any (bad) yellow leaves. Cut stems and leaves into 2-inch pieces, or smaller.
2. Peel kohlrabi and slice with a mandolin or cleaver. Combine sliced kohlrabi with stems and leaves. Set aside.
3. Salt kohlrabi, leaves, and stems, massage well and let sit for 30 minutes.
4. Next, rinse off salt, squeeze, and shake off all excess water. Place in a container that can handle boiling hot liquids.

   Bring Pickling Liquid to a full boil in a pot over high heat. Remove from heat and immediately pour over kohlrabi. Cover with plastic wrap. Make sure the wrap is flush across and pushed down onto the liquid surface so the veggies are completely submerged. Let cool to room temperature before refrigerating.

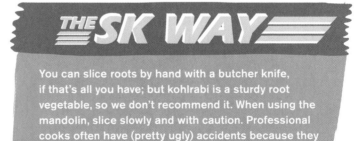

THE SK WAY

You can slice roots by hand with a butcher knife, if that's all you have; but kohlrabi is a sturdy root vegetable, so we don't recommend it. When using the mandolin, slice slowly and with caution. Professional cooks often have (pretty ugly) accidents because they slice too fast.

PICKLED MUSTARD GREENS

I'll happily admit that I got this idea after eating at the original Tsujita, one of LA's most famous ramen/*tsukemen* joints, with a common two-hour wait. Though I love their *tsukemen* and ramen, I love their chili pickled mustard greens even more. This is our version.

2–4 SERVINGS

1 pound Chinese mustard greens, cleaned and cut into 2-inch pieces

Kosher salt, for cleaning

6 garlic clove, crushed

1 whole dried Thai chili, cut lengthwise with seeds

2 cups Pickling Liquid (page 244)

BALLS OUT
40–80 SERVINGS

10 pounds Chinese mustard greens, cleaned and cut into 2-inch pieces

Kosher salt, for cleaning

60 garlic cloves, crushed

10 whole dried Thai chilies, cut lengthwise with seeds

5 quarts Pickling Liquid (page 244)

1. Liberally cover (both sides of) mustard green leaves with salt and let sit for 30 minutes.

2. Rinse greens well to remove salt, gently wring out excess water from leaves, then place in a container with garlic and Thai chili.

   Bring Pickling Liquid to a full boil in a pot over high heat, then pour over mustard greens. Cover with plastic wrap. Make sure the wrap is flush across and pushed down onto the liquid surface so the veggies are completely submerged. Let cool to room temperature before refrigerating.

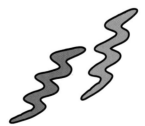

PICKLED PERSIAN CUCUMBERS

What's not to love about Persian cucumbers? Nothing. Not. A. Thing.

BALLS OUT
40–80 SERVINGS

20 medium Persian cucumbers, washed and sliced ⅛-inch thick

5 tablespoons whole cloves

5 tablespoons whole allspice

15 cups Pickling Liquid (page 244)

2–4 SERVINGS

2 medium Persian cucumbers, washed and sliced ⅛-inch thick

½ tablespoon whole cloves

½ tablespoon whole allspice

1½ cups Pickling Liquid (page 244)

Place cucumbers in a container that can handle boiling hot liquids. Add cloves and allspice.

Bring Pickling Liquid to a full boil in a pot over high heat. Remove from heat and immediately pour over cukes (aka cucumbers if you're like me and didn't know the shorthand for cucumbers even three years into the restaurant business—yes, I really am an idiot savant, I don't kid around about that). Cover with plastic wrap. Make sure the wrap is flush across and pushed down onto the liquid surface so the cukes are completely submerged. Let cool to room temperature before refrigerating.

PICKLED RED ONIONS

"Prett-ay"—Forest Gump . . . Oh wait, no, he said "Jenn-ay," which now has no relevance here. *face-palm*

BALLS OUT
40–80 SERVINGS

10 pounds red onion, thinly sliced

10 quarts Pickling Liquid (page 244)

2–4 SERVINGS

1 pound red onions, thinly sliced

4 cups Pickling Liquid (page 244)

Place onions in a container that can handle boiling hot liquids.

Bring Pickling Liquid to a full boil in a pot over high heat. Remove from heat and immediately pour over onions. Cover with plastic wrap. Make sure the wrap is flush across and pushed down onto the liquid surface so the veggies are completely submerged. Let cool to room temperature before refrigerating.

PICKLED SHREDDED CARROTS AND DAIKON

This is the most classic and iconic *Banh Mi* ingredient!

BALLS OUT
40–80 SERVINGS

5 pounds carrots, cleaned, peeled, and shredded

10 pounds Korean daikon radish (aka *lo bak*), cleaned, peeled, and shredded

Kosher salt, for cleaning

12½ quarts Pickling Liquid (page 244)

2–4 SERVINGS

½ pound carrots, cleaned, peeled, and shredded

1 pound Korean daikon radishes (aka *lo bak*), cleaned, peeled, and shredded

Kosher salt, for cleaning

5 cups Pickling Liquid (page 244)

1. Make sure both carrots and daikon are shredded to the same size while preparing. We like them less limp and a tad stiff, but still thin and crisp. Transfer to a bowl. Salt shredded veggies and massage well. Let sit for 30 minutes.

2. Next, rinse off salt, squeeze, and shake off all excess water. Place in a container that can handle boiling hot liquids.

   Bring Pickling Liquid to a full boil in a pot over high heat. Remove from heat and immediately pour over carrots and daikon. Cover with plastic wrap. Make sure the wrap is flush across and pushed down onto the liquid surface so the veggies are completely submerged. Let cool to room temperature before refrigerating.

PICKLED WATERMELON RINDS

Possibly better than the watermelon itself . . . no really . . . seriously . . . I'm still thinking about how definitive I feel that statement should be . . .

BALLS OUT
40–80 SERVINGS

Watermelon rinds (from an average 70+ pounds of watermelon), thinly sliced

Kosher salt, for cleaning

5 tablespoons Korean chili powder

1⅔ tablespoons whole cloves

20 bay leaves

5 tablespoons whole allspice

7½ quarts Pickling Liquid (page 244)

2–4 SERVINGS

Watermelon rinds (from an average 7+ pounds of watermelon), thinly sliced

Kosher salt, for cleaning

½ tablespoon Korean chili powder

½ teaspoon whole cloves

2 bay leaves

½ tablespoon whole allspice

3 cups Pickling Liquid (page 244)

1. Passionately salt and massage watermelon rinds in a bowl. Let sit for 30 minutes.
2. Next, rinse off salt and shake off all excess water. Place in a container that can handle boiling hot liquids. Add chili powder, cloves, bay leaves, and allspice.
3. Bring Pickling Liquid to a full boil in a pot over high heat. Remove from heat and immediately pour over watermelon. Cover with plastic wrap. Make sure the wrap is flush across and pushed down onto the liquid surface so the (delicious) rinds are completely submerged. Let cool to room temperature before refrigerating.

Let pickle for two to three days before eating. Thank us via Twitter and Instagram sooner rather than later.

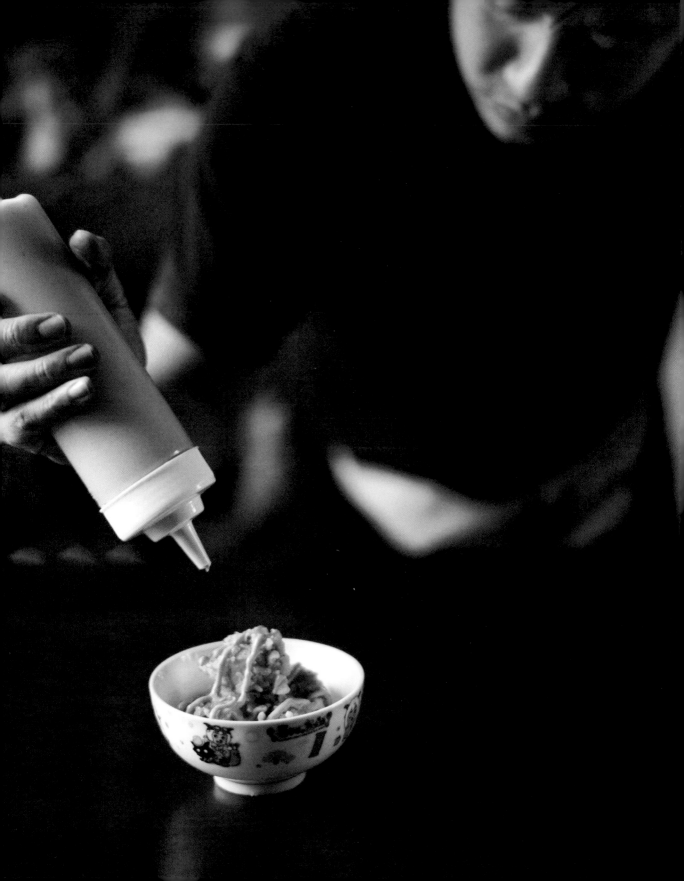

SPICY AIOLI

Ah-HAAAAAA! This is possibly the most important sauce to grace these pages, and the most important HALF of the Crispy Tofu Balls.

BALLS OUT
40–80 SERVINGS

7¾ quarts Starry Kitchen Mayo (page 254)

7⅓ cups sriracha sauce

½ teaspoon kosher salt

7 tablespoons sugar

3 cups minced garlic

9⅔ tablespoons lime juice

2–4 SERVINGS

2½ cups Starry Kitchen Mayo (page 254)

¾ cup sriracha sauce

1 pinch kosher salt

¾ tablespoon sugar

5 tablespoons minced garlic

1 tablespoon lime juice

Add Starry Kitchen Mayo to a bowl, fold in sriracha sauce, salt, sugar, garlic, and lime juice. In front of your very eyes, it should transform ("Oh MY!") into a nice solid orange—like our logo! If there are any streaks of yellow, you need to do a little more folding, and that's that. You've got our not-so-secret Spicy Aioli. It's easiest to store in a squeeze bottle, refrigerate, and squeeze onto your favorite foods or include on the side for dipping, like with Crispy Tofu Balls. HUZZAH!

STARRY KITCHEN MAYO

Quite a few recipes in this book include my personal "Oh WOW I didn't know you can do that!" anecdote. Making your own mayo, which I used to despise, is one of those instances.

BALLS OUT
40–80 SERVINGS

48 large eggs yolks

4 quarts plus
3¼ cups oil *

2–4 SERVINGS

5 large eggs yolks

2 cups oil *

* Any oil works, but choose wisely, because each kind of oil will change the flavor of your mayo. If you figure out some revelatory oil combo, let us know!

1. The basic instructions are to blend the yolks together first, then slowly introduce the oil in a steady stream. Do NOT pour the oil too quickly. If the mixture is more liquid than mayo emulsion, stop pouring oil and continue mixing. You might have a chance to recover before you get to the point of no return, which is to say, an oil and yolk that just won't emulsify.

2. There are four ways to do this (including the janky restaurant hack way). The first way, which is the hardest and most exhaustive, is how we used to make it when we started Starry Kitchen out of our apartment, followed by easier ways.

   MIX YOLKS IN A BOWL WITH A WHISK AND NOTHING ELSE. If you do this, don't even TRY to stream in the oil. Just add in a little bit of oil at a time, then mix until the oil is completely immersed in the mayo. When there's no visible layer of oil, add a LITTLE bit more oil. (So tired just thinking about this way.)

   MIX YOLKS IN A BOWL USING A HAND MIXER, with a constant start/stop stream of oil.

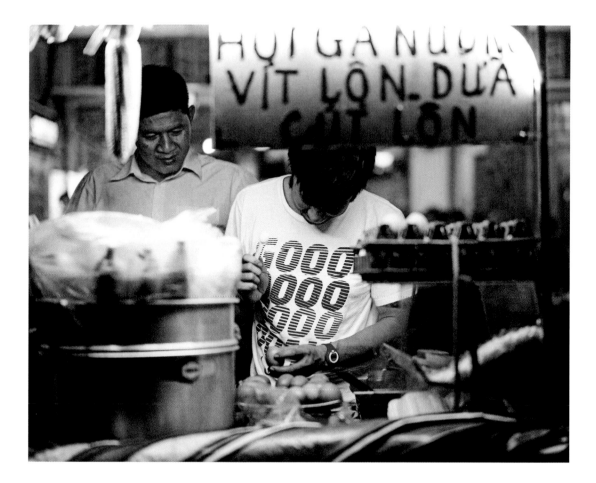

MIX IN A BOWL with a stand mixer. Run the mixer at a constant speed, allowing for the luxury of a slow, steady stream of oil.

THE JANKY WAY you probably won't read about in any other book is how we most often do it in the restaurant. Mix yolks with an industrial food processor—we use the Robot Coupe, the most common food processor in the business—and run the blades at maximum speed! Stream in oil slowly, and watch mayo magic happen.

SUPERCONCENTRATED CANTONESE CHICKEN STOCK

We use this chicken stock in a LOT of our dishes, and Asians don't go making diluted stocks like French cooks do, so our stock is made superconcentrated so that the water barely covers the bones in the process. The Starry Kitchen way is to engulf the kitchen with the aroma from the stock until you can SEE the flavor in the stock. And that ain't a joke or euphemism either—you can LITERALLY see it!

BALLS OUT

40–80 SERVINGS

10 pounds chicken breasts

10 pounds chicken wings*

10 quarts cold water

20 fresh ginger, cut into ¼-inch thick slices

10 stalk(s) scallions, cut into 1-inch pieces

6⅔ tablespoons Chinese cooking wine or sherry

FOR ADDED BODY:

10 (¼-ounce) packets unflavored gelatin

2½ cups cold water

2–4 SERVINGS

1 pound chicken breasts

1 pound chicken wings*

4 cups cold water

2 fresh ginger, cut into ¼-inch thick slices

1 stalk scallion, cut into 1-inch pieces

2 teaspoons Chinese cooking wine or sherry

FOR ADDED BODY (OPTIONAL):

1 (¼-ounce) packet unflavored gelatin

¼ cup cold water

* Any combination of chicken meat works, but we recommend this particular ratio for flavor and depth. Adjust to your liking, but remember, every little bit counts . . .

1. Rinse chicken under cold running water. Place chicken in a large pot, add water, and if the chicken is still exposed add more water to barely cover the chicken. DON'T use hot water to speed up the boiling process. Hot water straight from the tap leaves a distinctly artificial, technically "yucky," and cloudy flavor.

2. Add ginger, scallions, and rice wine. Bring to a boil over high heat, occasionally skimming off the gunky foam that rises to the top so you can rid your stock and the world of the impurities that will taint you and your stock.

3. Cover (with a tiny crack) and reduce heat. Simmer for 2 hours. Remove from heat and strain finished stock through a chinois, or fine-mesh strainer, into a large enough container or bowl.

4. If the stock doesn't have enough body to your liking, in a separate bowl mix unflavored gelatin with cold water, then mix with chicken stock.

5. Do not season! To make sweet and deep savory love to your mouth, hold off on seasoning the stock until the time is right. It is best left for

whatever wonderful recipe you're cooking. Each dish is seasoned with different savory elements in the place of salt, but you can get creative for your own recipes as long as you think of whatever you season it with as being a "salty" element = fancy mix-and-matching with something like kelp (aka *kombu*) or similar.

6. If storing for later, cool off stock uncovered until it is lukewarm or close to room temperature before storing in a refrigerator or freezer. If you're trying to be smart and think the fridge will cool off the stock for you, you're wrong and it may ruin other ingredients in your fridge because it will heat your fridge up instead and the stock will go bad because it wasn't cooled off properly.

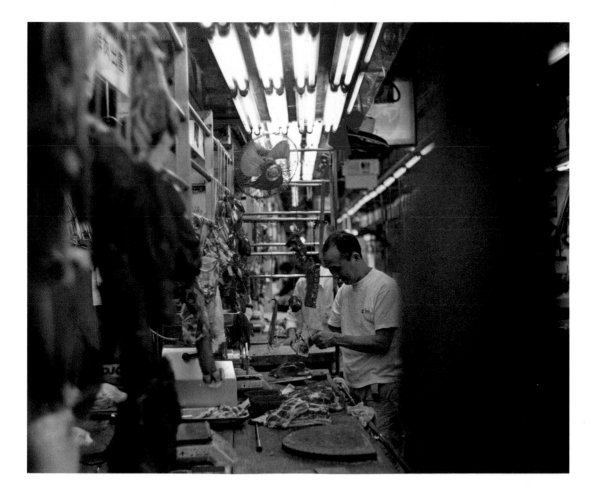

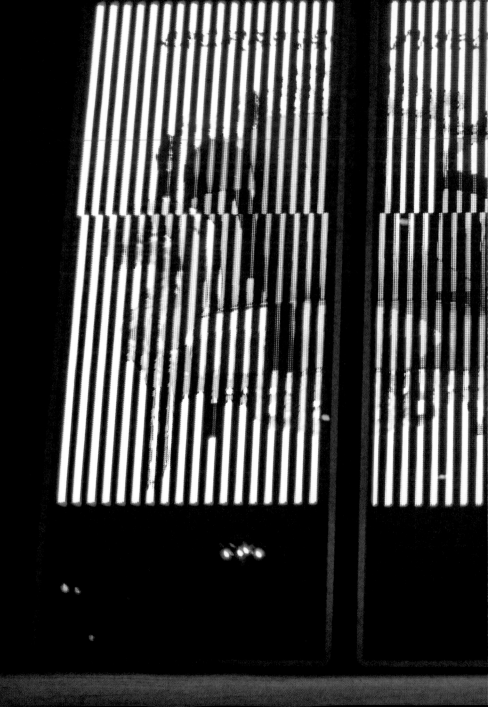

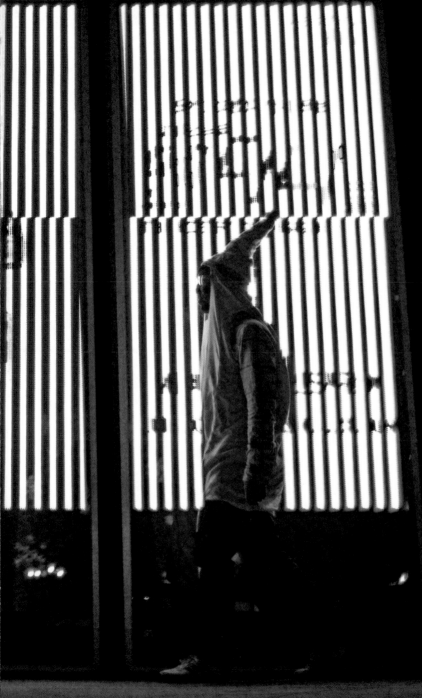

ACKNOWLEDGMENTS

I AM INDEBTED TO TOO MANY PEOPLE WHO HAVE HELPED ME OUT ALONG THE WAY TO NAME IN THE LIMITED SPACE HERE. BUT, FIRST AND FOREMOST, I WOULD LIKE TO THANK MY WIFE, THI, MY SPECIAL LADY, THE LOVE OF MY TUMULTUOUS LIFE, AND THE TRUE CULINARY FORCE BEHIND STARRY KITCHEN. I COULD NEVER HAVE SURVIVED THESE CRAZY-ASS ADVENTURES WITHOUT YOU— NOR WOULD I HAVE WANTED TO WITHOUT YOU BY MY SIDE (TOLERATING ME). AFTER READING MY BOOK, MANY PEOPLE WILL QUICKLY REALIZE HOW UNAPOLOGETICALLY ANNOYING I CAN BE, AND HOW THI SURPRISINGLY STILL LOVES ME. I WILL ALWAYS BE GRATEFUL FOR THAT.

I would also like to thank our parental units, Tuong Le and Tam Tran, and Dung and Suong Tran (no relation; I checked!)—we wouldn't be born without y'all! A big thanks, too, to my sister, Vivien Ly Jordan, and her misfit fam Jon Jordan (an accomplished author himself), young Zoë, and Rowan. Alan, John and Ken Tang—"Rock" beer forever. Many thanks to our OC fam, especially "Ba Noi," Hai, Hanh Nam, Kim, Khoi, Kiem, Frankie, Teresa, and . . .arrrrrgh . . . there are far too many to list!

Without the help and silent support of Marc R., Marimelle, Jerome and the entire Pascual Fam, including Dingane and Eric C, among a few others mentioned elsewhere, we literally wouldn't have gotten as far as we have. We are indebted to you, and paying you back that debt remains at the top of our minds.

A special shout-out to the numerous people who have helped us out at events, including but not limited to: Kemble Huang, Jin Nam, Rebekah Shibley, and Emily Lu. Our batch of "cute" 2011 interns: David Shu, Brian Leung, and Labobatory boba boss, Elton Keung. The Kickstarter crew: Jordan Gilbert, Heather Somaini, Tere Throenle, Julie Zwillich, Kellie Patry, Chris McIntosh, Nicholas Castelli, and David Vottero. The 766 just-as-crazy-as-us Kickstarter backers, including (but seriously not limited to) those craziest of $10,000 backers, Josh, Caroline T., and Julia H. Thankfully we didn't

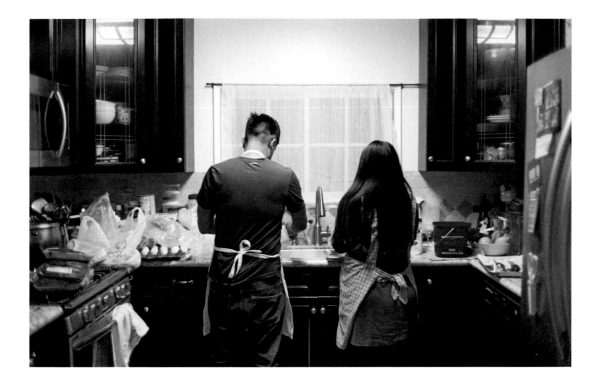

raise it all, so you guys were off the hook! *phew* haha. The multiple generations of Project-by-Project LA crew that still loves us even if I oft-times offend their guests, including Kevin Hsu, JT Kim, Lisa Thong. Shauna Dawson, Marcus Beer, Javier Cabral, and Paola Briseño. Christine Choi, just for being resilient. And our Mexicali Taco Crew: Esdras Ochoa, Javier Fregoso, Paul Yoo, Matt Kim, and Kristen Jue. Mexicali parking lot tacos FOREVER!

Thanks to the catalysts, Roger and Peter B. and Renee K, who inspired us to move on to crazier adventures.

For the seemingly unrecognized-but-not-forgotten help over the years, a big Starry Kitchen thank you to Brian "The Hair" Saltsburg, Abby Abanes. Jojo Subrata, Laura Osborne, Tim Hall, Richard Jun, and Byung Joo. Thanks, too, to the JACCC Crab Fest crew: Leslie Ito, Steven Wong, Helen Ota, Kisa, Janet Hiroshima, Kristin Fukushima, Gary Kawaguchi,

the crab cracking crew, and ALL the volunteers who continually lend their hands in this annual endeavor. I also want to acknowledge Craig "Wolvesmouth" Thornton, Julian Fang, Caleb Chen, and Sandra Kim, and Team "Mendo"—Mario del Pero, Ellen, Sean, and Chef Judy Han.

To Miss Heidi Starnes Barr, the Dallas/Carrollton gang—Jessy Jessy John, William Soo, Alex Soo, Tony Nguyen, Johnson Nguyen, and everyone else—my University of Texas at Dallas fam—Patty Atchley, Matt Grygar, Matt "Capitol" Hill, Anna Eisenmann, Tejal Shah, Jacob Gurwitz, Casey, and Mandy—and the rest! The Viet film *Wave*—Ham Tran, Stephane Gauger, Timothy Linh Bui, Kenneth Nguyen, Anderson Le, Jenni Trang Le, and Charlie Nguyen: From the bottom of my heart, thank you.

To Dylan Walker and the entire Walker clan: you are still my favorite ("fucking") Thanksgiving family.

Over the years, we've (luckily) received amazing

coverage from local and national media. At the risk of ruining their professional objectivity, I would like to give special thanks to Jonathan Gold, Amy Scattergood, Besha Roddell, Jenn Harris, Betty Hallock, Matt Kang, Kat Odell, Daniela Galarza, Leslie B. Suter, Leslie Balla, Elise McDonough, Jeff Miller, Alex Cohen, and Evan Kleiman, and everyone at KCRW's Good Food.

Laurent Quenioux taught me more about food and running a kitchen than anyone. Daniel Vasquez, Kevin Villegas, Drew, Christian, Debow, Helen "Striker" Springut, Daniel K Nelson, John Goldman, Zahra Bates, Sidney, Cindy and the Zerah fam, Nazie Shekarchi, Michaele Musel, Mark "Frosty" McNeil, all of Dublab, and all the other crazy pop-up and marijuana dinner crew . . . woo hoo!

Thanks, too, to all the LA chefs and operators we've worked with, sometimes pissed off, and have been inspired by, including Bruce Kalman, Chris Oh, Yong Kim, Ted Kim, Michael Voltaggio, Michael Fiorelli, Michael Cimarusti, Steve Samson, Zach Pollack, Kuniko Yagi, Pablo Moix, Steve Livigni, Alex Day, David Kaplan, Devon Tarby (I think I'm going to call you "Tarbs" from now on), Bill Chait, who even defended me from being trolled in a private food forum, Jason Park, Ludo and Krissy Lefebvre, Pawan and Nakul and Arjun Mehendro, Alvin Cailan, Charles Olalia, Josh Smith, and way too many others to name here!

Thanks to John Liu, Carley Lake, Cruz Resendez, Allen Narcisse and the huge UberEats crew, as well as Gabe Fawkes, Cindy Kim, Jordan Weiss . . . but really Tali Weiss—Team Button Mash . . . FOREVER!

Through everything Tim Kwok, Maya Lim, Meyuh Huynh, Dan Ding, Joeann, and Hai Tran amazingly stuck by our sides.

Bao Nguyen, you're the best-est photographer travel partner around.

To Marissa Patino, our first-ever employee who STILL works with us, and the countless others who have either loved or deplored working with us: There is NO Starry Kitchen without you guys.

Thanks to my old bosses, Chris Smith and Cassian Elwes! And of course Rena Ronson, Jerome Duboz and his better half, Margo Klewans, Casey Engelhardt, Emily Caitlin, and my many other former comrades "in the trenches" at WMA.

A special Balls Out thank you to Cameron Kadison, my agent Nicole Tourtelot, Kristina Sorensen, and just a few of my indie film crew: Tim and Karrie League, Michael Lerman, Dave Boyle, Mye Hoang, Rich Wong, Dusty, and H.P. Mendoza.

For my Underground supporters: Ava Green, Michelle Ko, Quan Phung, Chil Kong, Erin Quill, Alex Ow, Karin Anna Chung, Gloria Fan, Andy Pao, and so many more. Thank you. The Wick family "Cousins Club," Garlic noodle obsessive— Bryan Lee O'Malley and Hieu Ho.

Thanks to the early Chinatown crew: George Yu, Shirley, Amnaj, Roy Choi, ALIIIIIIIIIIIIIIIIIIIIIIIIIIICE, and Caroline Shin. And for the Italian restaurant owner who we THINK told on us and those two health department inspectors who tried to bust us—you were literally the catalyst that made us bigger.

Thank you mucho to my editor, Miles Doyle, for giving me, a confused Asian-American kid from Texas, this incredible first-world opportunity, and the entire (patient and tolerant) bicoastal HarperOne team in San Francisco and New York, including Lucy Albanese, Lisa Zuniga, Kim Dayman, Jane Chong, and Eva Avery, for helping me pull it off. Thank you, too, to Shubhani Sarkar for designing a truly amazing book and to my good friend Joseph Harmon for the book's stunningly cool cover and the equally cool illustrations dotted throughout the interior.

Finally, I want to thank ALL our fans—I still can't believe we have ANY fans!—the city of Los Angeles, our eclectically passionate eaters, as well as the chefs, cooking staff, proprietors, and waitstaff who have helped make LA the best food scene in the world. We are honored to be part of it.

INDEX

Page numbers in *italics* refer to illustrations.

French/Green/Long Beans, 187, *188–89*
Fried Chicken Waaaaaaaaaaaaangs, Double-, 46, *47,* 48
Fried Pork Chop, Taiwanese, 17–18
fried rice, 203; Galangal Chicken Fried Rice, 194–95; Roast Pork Belly XO Fried Rice, 202–3; Shrimp and Grilled Pineapple Fried Rice, 196–97; Spam Brussels Sprout Fried Rice, 192–93
Fried Steak, Chicken (aka Country Fried Steak), 233–34
"Fries," Curry Tofu, *188–89,* 190
Fritters, Five-Spice Apple (Formerly Known as Fluffy the Apple Fritter and Its Banana Jam Sidekick), 149–50
fruits. *See specific fruits*
funemployment, 225–34

Sauce, 49; Watermelon Ginger Agua Fresca, 138
Ginger Sesame Rainbow Roasted Carrots (aka Roasted Carrots with Sweet Soy Glaze), 139
Ginger Sesame Sake Sauce, 242
Goji Berries, Canto-Style Chayote, Enoki, and, 142
Gold, Jonathan, 108, 109
Good Ol' Omelet, *188–89,* 190
Grammar Rodeo, 108–9
Green Curry Silky Tofu, 94–95, *95*
green tea, 153; Green Tea Lemon Latte Cookies, 153–54
Green Tea Lemon Latte Cookies, 153–54
Grilled Beef Wrapped in Sesame Leaves (Bó Lá L´ôt), 89, *90,* 91
Grilled Fish Heads and Tails, 128–29, *129*
Grilled Pineapple Fried Rice, Shrimp and, 196–97
Grilled Pork Belly and Pork Patty, Hanoi (aka Bun Cha Hanoi), 167, *168,* 169
Grilled Turmeric Fish with Dill and Onion, Hanoi, 165–66, *166*
growing up Asian, 119–22
Guerrilla Tacos, 218
Gumbo, Singaporean Chili Crab, 222–23

heirloom vegetables, 139
High Times, 109
Hoison Peanut Dipping Sauce, 191
honey: Honey Bourbon Cream Sauce, 243; Honey Sesame Dressing, 45
Honey Bourbon Cream Sauce, 243
Honey Sesame Dressing, 45
Hong Kong, 155, 227, 228
hot pot, 63, 93
how to eat crab, *216–17*

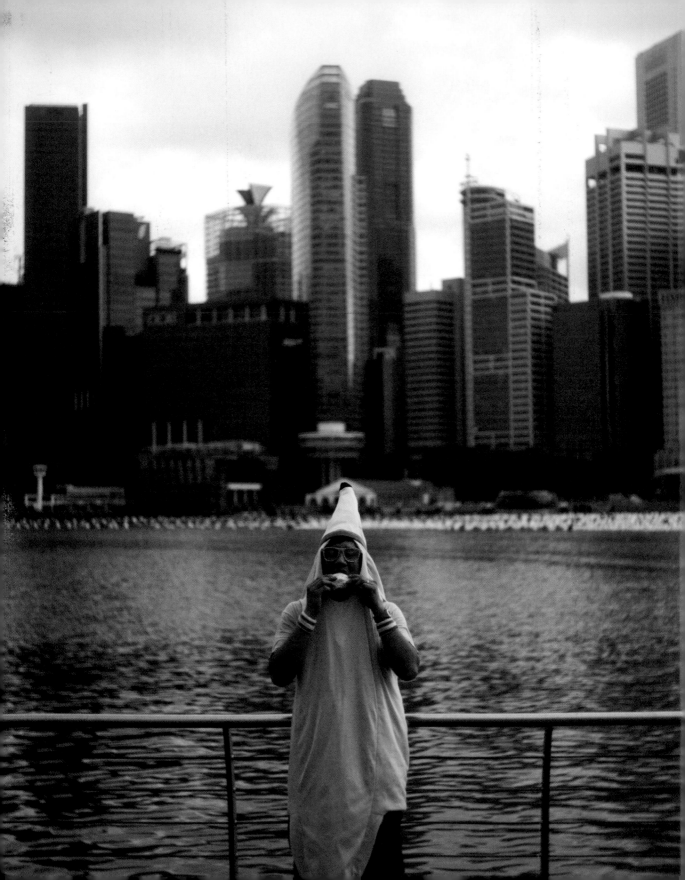